T0361861

Tomorrow I'll Be Slim

Why do so many people try dieting, only to fail? What distinguishes those who succeed from those who do not? Are fat people really any different from thin people? What makes us eat, and how do we stop eating? And how can dieting trigger problems with eating normally?

Originally published in 1989, Sara Gilbert discusses these questions in *Tomorrow I'll Be Slim*, and draws on what is known about the psychology of eating, overeating, and weight control to dispel a number of popular myths about dieting. She shows how unsuccessful dieting can lead to new problems with eating and weight control. She points out that long-term success in slimming has more to do with individual factors such as a dieter's expectations, self-confidence, or social and family circumstances than with 'will-power'; and as much to do with how a diet is managed as with the content of a diet sheet. She suggests ways in which people who want to be slimmer can make a realistic assessment of their need to diet. She explains how individuals who seriously need to lose weight or change the way they eat might draw up effective strategies for themselves and prepare for the inevitable difficulties we all face whenever we try to change old habits. Finally, she addresses the problems of taking the emphasis off dieting and examining our attitudes to a slim figure as the key to happiness itself.

Tomorrow I'll Be Slim

The psychology of dieting

Sara Gilbert

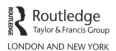
Routledge
Taylor & Francis Group

LONDON AND NEW YORK

First published in 1989
by Routledge

This edition first published in 2013 by Routledge
27 Church Road, Hove, BN3 2FA

Simultaneously published in the USA and Canada
by Routledge
711 Third Avenue, New York, NY 10017

Routledge is an imprint of the Taylor & Francis Group, an informa business

Publisher's Note
The publisher has gone to great lengths to ensure the quality of this reprint but
points out that some imperfections in the original copies may be apparent.

Disclaimer
The publisher has made every effort to trace copyright holders and welcomes
correspondence from those they have been unable to contact.

A Library of Congress record exists under ISBN: 0415028442

ISBN: 978-0-415-71254-5 (hbk)
ISBN: 978-1-315-88388-5 (ebk)

TOMORROW ~ I'LL BE ~ SLIM

THE PSYCHOLOGY OF DIETING

SARA GILBERT

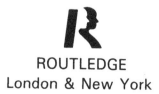

ROUTLEDGE
London & New York

First published in 1989 by
Routledge
11 New Fetter Lane, London EC4P 4EE
29 West 35th Street, New York NY 10001

© 1989 Sara Gilbert

Printed in 10/12 Times by Billing & Sons Ltd, Worcester

British Library Cataloguing in Publication Data

Gilbert, Sara
Tomorrow I'll be slim.
1. Physical fitness. Slimming. Diet.
Psychological aspects
I. Title
613.2'5'019
ISBN 0-415-02844-2

Library of Congress Cataloging in Publication Data

also available

ISBN 0-415-02844-2

CONTENTS

ACKNOWLEDGEMENTS

Figure 1 is reproduced from *Treat Obesity Seriously* by J.S. Garrow (1981) by permission of Churchill Livingstone.

Figure 2 is reproduced from 'Obesity: a report of the Royal College of Physicians', *Journal of the Royal College of Physicians of London* 17, 1, with the permission of the Royal College of Physicians.

The table in Chapter 7 is adapted from *The Great British Diet* by the British Dietetic Association and Dr Andrew Stanway (1985) and published by Century Hutchinson Ltd.

The weight chart in Chapter 8 (Figure 3) is reproduced by permission of the Health Education Authority, London.

The illustrations on pages 39 and 96 were supplied by Nicole Ryan.

A book about eating and weight must span many areas of specialist knowledge. Such a book could not be tackled by a single professional without access to the ideas and writings of many other people, both in the same and in different fields of work. I have been helped to clarify my thoughts in the area of diet and weight and about psychological research in general over the past few years both by the discussions I have had with colleagues and through reading about the ideas and work of other people with an interest in the area.

Among the people I should like to acknowledge personally are Dr Merrill Durrant, Dr Chris Frith, Professor Andrew Mathews, Professor Trevor Silverstone (for his suggestion that I write in the first place), and all my colleagues past and present in the Psychology Department at Northwick Park Hospital.

In particular I should like to thank Professor John Garrow for reading and commenting on part of this manuscript; Sue Crowther, dietitian, for her comments on Chapter 7; and Lucy Isenberg, Sally Johnson, and Vivien Korn for their willingness to read draft chapters and offer constructive criticism and advice. Ultimately, of course, the responsibility for any errors of fact is my own.

My thanks go also to the many patients who have shared with me their thoughts and often difficult and painful feelings around the topic of weight control.

On a more personal note, I should like to thank my husband Nicholas, for always making himself available to read first drafts and offer comments; he deserves particular thanks for his support and forbearance while I wrote two books, an activity which is punctuated alternately by periods of inactivity, periods of worry, and periods of strict seclusion.

Sara Gilbert

INTRODUCTION

Most books which discuss diets make promises. They suggest that if you follow this diet, eat that food, cook in such a way, you are guaranteed to lose weight and enjoy a healthy life. This book promises none of those things.

People who are seriously overweight are no longer the only people who diet. Ever increasing numbers of people, women in particular, are worrying about their weight and trying to control what they eat. Yet, dieting does not always produce the rewards that slimmers are looking for; it often creates new problems with weight and eating for dieters and their families. For slim people and fat people alike, problems with overeating and dieting are reaching epidemic proportions.

Dieters often blame themselves for these problems, perhaps because of certain commonly held assumptions which imply that successful dieters have something that other people do not have. They believe that successful dieters have 'will-power', for example, or stronger personalities, than people who 'allow' themselves to become fat and fail repeatedly to lose weight by dieting. They forget that very many fat people have tremendous control over their lives: holding responsible jobs, being creative and competent in many spheres; and that it is only in relation to dieting that they 'fail'. What then do we mean by failure in dieting, and is it indeed the person who has failed, or is there something wrong with dieting itself or with the expectations we are putting on ourselves to eat in a certain way?

It has become increasingly clear over the past few years that most diets fail because dieting itself is an imperfect way to lose weight and maintain the loss. The temperament of dieters, their attitude

1

towards a particular regime, their style of coping with life's stresses, together with the way in which the diets are designed and administered: all these aspects influence each other and may be as crucial for success as the composition of the diet-sheet itself.

This book is not primarily about diets, calories, or food. It is an attempt to piece together what is known about the psychology of eating, overeating, and weight control, in a way that might make sense to anyone contemplating going on a diet or worried about their weight. It examines the psychological differences between fat and thin people, and between those who are able to diet and those who are not. It discusses the causes of overeating and the psychological effects of dieting. As a result of reading this book I hope that would-be dieters will have a better understanding of what makes us eat or not and of the ways in which dieting can affect us. I hope too that after reading this book, anyone with a diet or weight problem might have a clearer understanding of what is causing the problem and will be able to work out for themselves a way to alter their diet or lose weight permanently. Above all, my aim in this book is to provide information which will suggest ways of becoming less concerned about weight and diet both for people who seriously need to alter their diet or lose weight and for those who do not.

The idea for this particular book began to grow eight years ago, when I had just started to work in the Nutrition Department of the Clinical Research Centre in Harrow. I was involved in running a research project, the aim of which was to find out the best way to treat obesity on an outpatient basis. As the psychologist on the project, it was my job to run a series of behaviour therapy groups to teach people how they could change their eating habits. In order to do this properly I needed to give people information about specific strategies they might use both to identify their main problems and to make difficult changes. I wrote a treatment manual for use in the groups, based on some ideas which had proven fairly successful in the United States. It was at this stage that it began to seem like a good idea to write a book which could be useful not only to patients in a clinic but also to anyone who had a weight problem. There certainly was a need for something on the British market, but although the ideas on which I was basing my research were by now fairly well established, I still did not know how well they would work in practice, here in the National Health Service.

At first, the results of my own work were discouraging. The most startling result of our outpatient study, which took in over a hundred people in one year, was its very high drop-out rate. There was no point in writing a book about any brilliant new treatment if most of the people to whom it was offered simply lost interest after the first few weeks of the programme. Perplexed, I attended conferences and symposia on obesity and listened to the results of other studies. I met a colleague who worked in a clinic similar to mine. To our mutual relief, we discovered that our experiences had been almost identical. We were both putting into practice techniques that had proven fairly successful in the academic papers we had read but which in our hands might just as well have been conjured up on the spot for all the good they were doing any of the overweight people we were working with.

I began to investigate the research literature for clues as to the partial failure of our project. It became clear that no one research study has thrown up all the answers. However, an extensive search through all the papers on diets, and on differences between fat and thin people, dieters and non-dieters, reveals that there are certain common factors which lead to dieting success or failure, and which have very little to do with the nature of the diet itself.

In these pages I have summarized those findings. I have combined them with the experience I have gained through working with dieters of all weights in order to make some suggestions as to how an eating or weight problem might be tackled.

In writing this book I have necessarily simplified what is known. However, the results of academic research rarely give clear-cut answers, and there is always some measure of interpretation which goes into reporting them. There is even more room for interpretation when it comes to extrapolating from the results of several studies to explain the way things are in the real world and it is difficult always to be entirely objective. This is why those enticing covers that suggest the end to all your diet problems, that advertise this new diet or that new way of eating or cooking, can never tell the full story; they can only beguile us into trying yet one more method: a method which might have its successes but which inevitably also has its casualties. In this book I shall try not to pretend that there are any simple answers: only to report what is known, and to make some attempt to draw the disparate ideas into some meaningful whole so that readers can have the chance to decide for themselves what might, and what might not work for them personally.

No doubt my own biases will appear, but ultimately I hope that you, the reader, will be able to draw your own conclusions.

Chapter One

A BOOK WITHOUT
A PROMISE

Most serious dieters have lost count of the new diets they have read about in magazines and newspapers. Many of these diets are a variation on a theme; nearly all promise immediate success. So popular is diet news that it is an easy matter to obtain media coverage on almost any novel idea, however trivial. Often on a Sunday, a quality newspaper devotes space to reporting the launch of a new diet such as the 'Champagne diet', claimed by its author to have fat-metabolizing properties which help to speed weight loss.[1]

The sad truth is, however, that fat cannot be shed quickly: rapid weight loss means losing part of a temporary store and a great deal of water, and is rarely permanent. Anyone who needs to lose more than a few pounds in weight will have to think in terms of weeks, perhaps even months, rather than days.

How is it then that so many of us are beguiled, time and time again, into buying a new magazine, trying a new diet, or joining a new slimming club? The myth of the miracle diet has a magnetic pull, and if it is truly unworkable, how does it survive?

One answer to this question may lie in the nature of the group of people who diet and their reasons for doing so.

PEOPLE WHO DIET

Up to one-third of men and women in the western world are said to be overweight (see Chapter 2). However, the number of people who see themselves as overweight is twice that of people who actually do weigh more than they should. More normal-weight women than men believe themselves to be overweight. Moreover, not only do these normal-weight people believe they weigh too much: many also worry about their weight or have lives that are in some way restricted by it.[2]

In this context, dieting is extremely common, and it is not only the fatter people who try to lose weight. In 1980–1 Dr Jeffery and his colleagues from the Epidemiology department of the University of Minnesota carried out a survey of some 2,000 men and women living in the town of Minneapolis. According to the people they questioned in the survey, 72 per cent of women and 44 per cent of men had tried dieting. By no means all of these people were fat, however, and the figures included 63 per cent of women and 22 per cent of men *who had never been overweight*.[3] The results of other surveys have also supported this finding: that many people, women in particular, mistakenly believe themselves to be overweight, and that at least every other woman who is not overweight has tried dieting. Indeed, only half of the women who went to slimming clubs in Minneapolis actually met objective criteria for being overweight (see Chapter 2).

Thus, the prevalence of dieting is very high. Large numbers of people diet, often with little objective need.

There are more than 230 books on the subject of diet and slimming for the general reader currently in print.[4] The increase in the popularity of dieting over the past twenty years is reflected in a large increase in the circulation of magazines devoted to slimming. In 1966 there were no such magazines in Britain; in 1986 there were ten. The combined circulation of the seven magazines for which figures were available in the first half of 1986 was just under 777,000. In comparison, the joint circulation of the two magazines which have survived since 1976 was just under 377,000 in early 1976.[5] What the figures do not tell us, of course, is how far the increase in the figures can be explained by individuals buying more than one magazine now rather than by more people in general buying slimming magazines. Either way, however, it is clear that diet news is increasingly marketable.

The question that arises is how far is dieting actually effective, and related to this, how do people learn what to do?

HOW DO PEOPLE LEARN HOW TO DIET?

The second part of the question is more easily answered than the first. Most people diet on their own without recourse to professional or formal help. By far the majority of people trying to diet use a low-calorie regime according to both Dr Jeffery's survey in Minneapolis in 1981 and a *Which?* magazine survey in Britain in 1978.[6] The next most popular method reported by the *Which?* survey was a combination of diet and increasing normal exercise, such as walking to work. Very many people also try fasting, or other very low-calorie diets. The majority of these people get their information about what to do from magazines and newspapers;[7] and the next most common sources of information are friends and relatives.[8] A very large number of people also enrol in formal weight loss programmes such as a commercial slimming club. Forty per cent of dieters in the British (*Which?* magazine) survey and one in five women in the American survey had tried this method.

DOES DIETING WORK?

As far as success is concerned, magazine and newspaper articles on the subject of dieting are largely optimistic. They may suggest that dieting is often difficult and that it can take a long time to achieve results, but they imply that it is rarely impossible, that anyone can do it if they try hard enough.[9] In actual fact they have little evidence on which to base such an assumption, as no one really has a clear idea of how well people do when they try either dieting on their own or using a commercial club. It is not uncommon for the inventor of a new diet or the author of a book advertising a particular method to make extravagant claims for the diet's efficacy. Anyone can report that hundreds of people have tried a certain method and lost weight permanently. They can also publish letters purportedly received from successful customers. They know that most people have no way of checking to see whether the claim is true or the 'letters' genuine.

It would be cynical to assume that most people extolling the virtues of their particular brand of diet are in the business of deceiving the public, and it is likely that many of the individual comments published in praise of some diets are entirely genuine. However, it is important to remember that for every person who enjoys a particular product there may be another, or perhaps tens of people, who found no use for it at all or were in some way harmed by it. For every three people who succeed with the pineapple diet, the apple diet, or the five chocolate bars a day diet, there may be another three hundred who find the diets entirely useless.

Asking the dieters

If we wanted to find out how successful people are when they try dieting on their own, we would have to launch an almost impossible survey. First, we would have to select a large enough group of people to be representative of the population at large, including people of all ages, both sexes, and all levels of financial, educational, and occupational status. Having done this, we would have to catch them just at the time they had decided to go on a diet. We would have to weigh them and judge how overweight they were in relation to their height, and we would then have to catch them again at the end of their diet, which as anyone who has tried dieting knows could be anywhere between one day and one year or more. We would then have to weigh them again, and follow them up at a later stage, say in six months, one year, or even five years' time in order to find out how successful they had been at both losing the weight in the first place and keeping it off in the long term.

An alternative to this fairly laborious task would be to find a group of people who have tried dieting in the past and ask them how they got on with it. This too has its problems, as most of us have a very poor memory for fine details such as exactly what we used to weigh, how long the diet took, and just how many times we tried. In practice, however, it is a method that has been tried by a few researchers.

Stanley Schachter, an American psychologist interested in the subject of obesity, carried out his own survey, interviewing a total of 161 people including eighty-three current members of the Psychology department at Columbia University in 1977, and seventy-eight people living in a small seaside town.[10] In the interview, he asked people about their weight history from childhood onwards, and probed with more questions about any attempts to lose weight. Out of the 161 people interviewed forty-six had at some stage in their lives been overweight, and of these forty had tried dieting. Of these, twenty-five (just over two-thirds) reported that they had succeeded in losing weight and had managed to maintain weight losses of twenty-nine to thirty-nine pounds for several years. This sounds fairly optimistic; but the problem with the survey is that it was very small and may not be truly representative of the population at large. In Dr Jeffery's much larger survey in which he reported on interviews with over 2,000 people only one-third of dieters reported having achieved success.[11] Of course, the major problem with surveys of this kind is that we have only people's self-report to go on. In Dr Jeffery's survey, men reported themselves as having been more successful at dieting than the women. However, very many of the women who dieted were not overweight in the first place, so that the word 'success' in this context presents problems as we do not know how many of the dieters actually needed to lose weight.

Commercial slimming clubs

Another way of examining how successful people are at dieting is to consider what happens to people who join commercial slimming clubs. Up to forty per cent of female dieters try going to a club at some stage, which represents a fairly high proportion of dieters. In Britain, nearly 100,000 people attend weekly meetings of slimming clubs run by organizations such as Weight Watchers, *Slimming* magazine, and Silhouette.[12] About 10,000 of these people, that is one in ten people, are said to reach their target weight. Unfortunately, it is difficult to interpret the meaning of these figures as the clubs do not keep records on a national scale. Many of the 100,000 recruits could be people who rejoin some weeks after leaving in order to give the diet another try. This would render the figure of one in ten fairly optimistic (it might really be one in ten tries rather than one in ten people).

Whether people manage to reach their target or goal weight is, of course, a matter which may be less important than whether they manage to lose weight at all. Surveys in Britain, Scandinavia, and the United States have estimated that people who do not drop out of programmes early achieve a net loss of between 9.5 and 26 pounds (4.3 and 11.8 kilograms) on average, attending their clubs for an average time of between four and thirty weeks. While these figures include both people who have gained and people who have lost weight, they are not entirely unsatisfactory as clearly there are some initially very overweight people who are able to lose a significant amount of weight.

There is a major question mark, however, over the fate of those people who do not either lose a large amount of weight or achieve the target set for them by their club. It may be that some of them would prefer to continue attending in the hope that they will make further progress at a later stage; but in the words of Audrey Eyton, founder of Weight Watchers in Britain, 'Most commercial slimming groups, as they learn by experience, tend to toughen up their policy with strictures like "shed so much in a month or you'll get expelled"'.[13] If indeed clubs are putting pressure on their slow losers to leave the fold, this would have the effect of biasing the figures in the direction of greater success.

Many slimming club members drop out before they have reached goal weight. The numbers of people who do so are bound to vary from one club to another, but in one study in the United States half of the 108 women in one commercial programme had dropped out by six weeks, and 70 per cent by the twelfth week.[14] Dropping out of a programme would not have any significance if we knew that once having been to a slimming club most people had learned how to diet and were able to continue following the programme on their own at home. Most dieters, however, are unfortunately not able to do this. In one study of an Australian organization, the authors managed to follow up 131 out of 172 people who enrolled in a twelve-week programme, six months after the end of the programme.[15] Just over half the people who were prepared to fill in a questionnaire at this stage admitted to having gained weight again, and this of course casts doubt on the fate of those people who did not return their questionnaires.

What then of the people who do manage to lose a significant amount of weight? The authors of one survey in Britain sent questionnaires to 136 members of three slimming clubs who were known to have lost 14 pounds (6.3 kilograms) or more. Ninety-two people (just over two-thirds) replied. Twenty-two people (about a quarter) had regained all their lost weight and some of these had gained even more; fifty-eight people (nearly two-thirds) had regained some but not all of the lost weight; and only twenty-two people (13 per cent) had maintained their losses or managed to continue losing.[16]

There are some people then who manage, either on their own or with the help of a slimming club, to lose weight. A small proportion of these people lose a large amount of weight. Some people can sustain quite substantial losses for a considerable period of time; but these people are not in the majority. Many people are unable to stay in their club or on the diet long enough to lose a significant amount of weight. Others find that when they have left their club, or gone off the diet, the weight begins to creep back on again.

PROFESSIONAL HELP

If dieting on one's own or with the help of a slimming club fails, what alternatives are there for the would-be slimmer? One person to whom many people go for advice is their doctor or general practitioner (GP). Over half of the slimmers in the *Which?* magazine survey had at some stage talked to their GPs about losing weight, and they were more likely to have done so if they were dieting for health reasons than if they were dieting for the sake of their appearance. The kind of advice that is available from a GP will depend on the level of interest and expertise that particular doctor has. One GP has examined the dieting success of 204 patients in his practice, and found that of fifty-seven people who had lost more than 20 pounds (9.1 kilograms) at some time, thirty-eight had maintained this loss for at least five years.[17] However, by no means all GPs have an interest in helping people with their diets, and more than one-third of the people in the *Which?* survey who had consulted their GPs said that they were not particularly helpful.

Drug treatment

Half of the women in the *Which?* survey who consulted their GPs about their diet were offered drugs to help them lose weight. It has been estimated that the use of anorectic or appetite suppressant drugs costs the National Health Service some £4,000,000 per year.[18] The drugs used have the effect of making the user feel less hungry, or satisfied more quickly after eating. Amphetamines were used initially but are never advised now because of their stimulant effect on the central nervous system, leading to addiction in many cases. Drugs used nowadays are seen as being less dangerous either because they have a less stimulant action, for example diethylpropion (apisate/tenuate), or because they have a different way of working altogether, for example fenfluramine (ponderax). Nevertheless, patients have reported experiencing side effects with all of them to a varying degree, including difficulty with sleeping, nervousness, dry mouth, lethargy, and constipation;[19] and a few people are known to have become dependent on diethylpropion.

The extent to which appetite suppressing drugs help people to lose weight is fairly doubtful. In the short term, some research studies have shown that people can lose a few more pounds over a period of a few weeks when treated with drugs than with diet alone. However, as with other methods, individual responses vary in that some people do better with drugs, some do not.[20] Moreover, it is known that many people who are given pills by their doctor do not actually take them, and this raises the question of why people who are given drugs should in fact lose weight any faster than those who are not. Nevertheless, however effective they may be in the short term, drugs to reduce appetite are not a long-term solution to the problem of dieting. As soon as people stop taking them, the weight begins to creep back up again, particularly in people who have not learned any alternative practical strategies for eating less in the mean-time.

Seeing a dietitian

As an alternative to continuing to see patients themselves, many GPs refer to dietitians for advice. While dietitians are usually more able to give detailed dietary advice, the success of their treatment will depend partly, just as does the GP's, on their individual level of interest, and on how good the dieter is at following the prescribed diet. In fact the rate of drop-out from outpatient diet clinics is very high. Where attendance has been recorded, more than half the clients enrolled have dropped out within a few weeks. On the other hand, people who return to the clinics do manage to lose weight on the whole, usually at the rate of about a pound a week over six months.[21]

'ALTERNATIVE' METHODS OF WEIGHT LOSS

In view of the common difficulties experienced by many people in losing weight, it is not surprising that many people seek alternative solutions to the problem, some of which border on the magical. For example, many people who have tried the slimming clubs, their GP, dietitians, and failed, make the assumption that there is some fault with their psyche and that what they need is for will-power to be magically instilled into their minds. For such people, the pull of hypnosis is strong. In fact there is only a very limited scientific literature relating to hypnotherapy for weight reduction which does not support the idea that it is any more effective, or even as effec-tive, as other methods. Unfortunately all too many people are beguiled by the advertisements in the personal columns of newspapers and magazines into spending large amounts of money on 'treatment' meted out by people often with entirely bogus qualifications.[22] As a rule of thumb it is useful to remember that in Britain most qualified professionals are bound by a code of conduct drawn up by their professional associations not to advertise themselves in such a way as to make claims to being able to do things that are beyond their competence. This being the case, you should take any claims to cure smoking, overeating, shyness, and so on with a very large pinch of salt. If in doubt about a potential therapist's credentials ask your general practitioner, who should at least know what qualifications would be required by the National Health Service.

There is no foolproof solution to the weight loss dilemma. For some people it is clear that weight is not itself the issue at stake; for there are all too many people trapped in a cycle of dieting who have no need to be there at all. For others, it may be vital for their health to lose weight but the task itself is beset with problems. The person who succeeds with a diet is, contrary to many media messages, in the minority. There are far more people who have tried dieting and failed than there are people who have aspired to and achieved the sylph-like figure of the advertisements.

WHY DO SOME PEOPLE SUCCEED WHERE OTHERS FAIL?

Anyone reading this book may by now have acquired a fairly pessimistic view of the prospects of the would-be dieter. Certainly no promises have been made about foolproof methods, diets to end all diets. However, there is a positive aspect to the problem. This is that there are some people who do lose weight by dieting, with or without help; and some of these people maintain their losses for many years. It would be tempting to make the assumption that people who do well do so for one of two reasons: either because they have found the perfect diet, or because they are people who are imbued with a magical quality, an iron will that sustains them against all temptation. In fact, neither of these two explanations stands up very well to examination.

The perfect diet

Many different ways of dieting have been recommended by different people at different times. Diets may be low in fat, low in calories, low in carbohydrates, or high in fibre. Some diets consist of a series of set menus for particular meals and these diets vary in the degree to which they make sensible recommendations. Other diets consist of lists of foods to be eaten freely, eaten in moderation or avoided as far as possible (traffic light or no-counting diets). In addition there are starvation diets, which consist of eating very little for as long as possible and which for reasons to be discussed in Chapter 6 should be avoided.[23] According to the *Which?* magazine survey, more than half the slimmers who had tried a calorie controlled diet thought that it was the best method for long-term weight loss; and more than a quarter of people who tried them thought no-counting diets, low carbohydrate diets, and eating less in general were the best method.[24] There are some diets which are no good for anyone on health grounds, for example starvation diets or diets which restrict intake to one or two types of food. In relation to the 'perfect diet' however, we know that several people can start off on the same diet and while some will be able to keep to it, others will fail; some will lose weight, others will not.

'Will-power'

As for the 'will-power' concept, we all know people who are well organised, who drive themselves to work hard and who have many great achievements to be proud of. Yet these very same people, who can work although tired, who crowd more than seems humanly possible into twenty-four hours, may not be able to diet.

There was a time, not long ago, when man could not fly. At first, he said to himself 'If only I had wings; then I could fly'. There came a time when he saw that merely wishing for the impossible would not get him anywhere. Gradually he began to learn about the conditions that allow airborne creatures to fly, and hence to see how he could build a machine that would allow him to fly as if indeed he did have wings. Similarly, given the right conditions, there may be no reason why everyone who needs to should not be able to diet and lose weight.

A frequent result of not achieving a diet goal is that the dieter interprets the failure as a sign to 'try harder' next time. In practice this means saying to oneself something like this: 'I must be strong, I must try harder to resist (whatever food or situation is seen as that person's downfall) next time.' Trying harder usually means being somehow stronger willed, more resistant to temptation, and implies that there is only one factor which determines the success or failure of a diet.

The evidence suggests, however, that there are also several other factors, acting from both within and outside the person, that influence dieting outcome.

The presentation of a diet

A simple example of this is what happens to certain people when they diet under the guidance of a professional. One major difference between doctors seen as helpful and those seen as unhelpful by people who responded to the *Which?* survey was that satisfied patients were three times more likely than unsatisfied patients to have been asked to report back at regular intervals.[25] Mrs Smith, when given a diet to follow by her GP in Surrey, may fail miserably. She may on the other hand, upon moving to Northampton, be given a similar diet sheet by her new GP and do very well. Mrs Jones might attend a slimming club in Bristol and lose a few pounds, only to put them on again within the next few months. Upon moving to Manchester she might rejoin the club at a different branch, or join a different organization, lose eighteen pounds and maintain the loss for two years or more.

These kinds of differences cannot always be explained by sudden injections of 'will-power'. There are several reports of programmes where people assigned to dieting under one condition fare better than another, similar, group of people, assigned to a diet where the nutritional features are the same, but where the diet is administered in a different way. In recent years, for example, an increased success rate has been claimed consistently in programmes which teach some of the techniques derived from the group of psychological treatments known as 'behaviour therapy'. One group of researchers in Norway followed up members of a slimming club for five years.[26] In contrast to the findings in the British survey cited above,[27] only 15 per cent of the dieters reported that they had regained all of their lost weight after four years. It is unlikely that Norwegian dieters have any built-in initial advantage over British dieters. In fact, although individual group leaders worked in different ways, there are certain characteristics that all the Norwegian groups had in common, and which may have been absent in the British groups. These include: organizing members into small groups, the use of reward systems, and an emphasis on total changes in life-style in order to support the diet. There is also some evidence that people in groups lose more weight the more highly trained their therapists are in teaching people how to change their behaviour.

Sometimes the reasons for the improved success rate of one group of people in comparison with a similar group are less clear. For example, in our own study of outpatients, the people who were offered drug treatment attended the clinic for longer and lost on average more weight than people offered other treatments; but many of these people did not actually take their pills, which suggests that there may be something more subtle going on than a crude difference between two treatments on offer. There may be a complex interaction between the nature of a diet treatment on the one hand, and the way in which the dieter sees the situation and the likelihood of success on the other. This aspect of the attitude of dieters and the level of belief in their ability to diet is of course an area which has for many years exposed them to the manipulations of the media and a range of diet 'quacks'. There is often no limit to what a desperate person will pay in the faint hope of solving a chronic and intractable problem. Yet if only dieters could understand what it is about a particular diet offer that helps them to believe in and keep to the diet then they could use this very same aspect to their own advantage.

Differences between people

There are also differences in ability to diet between one person and another, apart from the differences intrinsic to treatment methods. There are many explanations for these differences other than that of 'will-power'. A dieter's attitude, borne of past success or failure, is only one of these. Some people would suggest that 'personality' may have something to do with ability to diet, and while this is not strictly true, certain aspects of the way in which we experience the world can influence individual dieting success or failure.

Besides the differences between us, there are also certain other factors which affect all of us to some degree. For example, the kind of food we eat and the way in which we eat it can affect our appetite and have a bearing on how easy or difficult it is for us to diet in any particular situation.

The purpose of this book is to explore some of these factors. The following chapters will examine diet programmes and the way they are administered on the one hand and differences between individuals and their response to dieting on the other. With these aims in mind, there will of course be little opportunity for making promises. If, however, we can have some understanding of what influences the way we eat, both in the normal course of events and when we are trying to diet, then we all stand a better chance of making informed decisions about whether to diet in the first place and of achieving success if we do.

Before we can begin to consider the problems of diets, dieting and fat people, it is important to establish what the need is for dieting in the first place. We know that there are large numbers of people, women in particular, who diet without apparently needing to. Who then are the people who do need to diet, and what determines their need? If indeed there are people who diet unnecessarily, why is it that losing weight is a matter of such crucial importance?

Chapter Two

WHY DIET?

Many people feel the need to diet. Their reasons for doing so may seem fairly understandable: to improve health; to be fashionable; and even to feel satisfied with a hard-won achievement. Yet successful dieting is elusive, and this raises two questions. First, how far is dieting a necessity and for whom; and second, where dieting is not essential to health, why has it come to hold a place of such great importance in the lives of so many?

A QUESTION OF HEALTH

The health reason for losing weight is the one that is perhaps most difficult for us to assess without professional help, mainly because there is so much controversy around the subject even in the medical world. Good health in general is fostered by many different factors. It depends on what we consume, including both what we eat and drink in the way of nutrients, and also of man-made substances such as alcoholic drinks, cigarettes, and other drugs. It depends also on how much exercise we take, on hereditary factors, the kind of work we do, and how stressful our lives are, at home and at work; it depends even on the nature of the very air we breathe. To a large extent, therefore, we rely for good health on a combination of luck, in relation to where we live and who our parents are, and self-control in the face of all the temptations that modern living offers us. We cannot change the way we are built; not many people move from one environment to another merely to avoid the effects of pollution, and few of us have the wisdom to see when our circumstances are proving too stressful to us, let alone have the courage to change them.

18

The question of good health, then, is a very complex one. It is an area of medicine which does not lend itself easily to exact assessment, and therefore forecasting what will happen to the health of any one of us over time is problematic.

Most of the medical research which revolves around this process of trying to predict good health or how long people might expect to live, is based on looking at single major factors, such as life stress, or how much a person smokes, or obesity.

WHAT IS OBESITY?

If we say that someone is obese, we imply by definition that they are too fat for the good of their health. 'Obesity is a condition in which energy stores, mainly fat, are too large.'[1] In an ideal world, we would be able to say how obese a person is based on the average ideal weight in their part of the world, taking into account local factors such as quality of diet and presence or absence of famine.[2]

In fact, obesity is defined numerically, in terms of the relationship between an individual's weight on the one hand, and his or her height on the other.[3]

The most widely used definition of obesity relates to the Metropolitan Life Insurance Tables, published in 1960 and revised in 1979.[4] These tables are based on data collected from people wanting to take out life assurance policies in the United States and they provide a range of weights for males and females of different heights. A person who weighs more than 20 per cent over the upper limit of weight for their height is considered to be obese.[5]

Another way of defining obesity is to use a calculation called the Body Mass Index (BMI). This means dividing a person's weight (in kilograms) by the square of their height (in metres). The desirable range for men is 20 to 25, and that for women is 20 to 24. Anyone with a BMI of between 25 and 30 would be considered overweight, and above 30, obese.[6]

A British consultant in nutrition, Professor John Garrow, has used this information to create a table which is easy to use, and which divides weight categories into four – normal, slightly overweight, moderately obese, and grossly obese (see Figure 1).

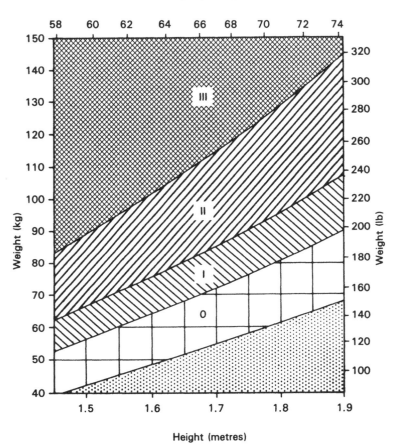

Source: Treat Obesity Seriously, J.S. Garrow, 1981

Figure 1 Relation of weight to height defining the desirable range (0) and grades I, II and III obesity, marked by the boundaries $W/H^2 = 25-29.9$, $30-40$, and over 40 respectively.

HOW OVERWEIGHT ARE WE?

Estimates of the number of people who are obese vary. Taking all the estimates together, obesity has been estimated to affect up to one-third of the populations of the United States and Britain.[7] The prevalence of obesity increases with age, up to about age 60, after which people become lighter. Thus, between five and twenty children and adolescents in every hundred are overweight; by the time they reach their mid-20s, according to a Report of the Royal College of Physicians, 31 per cent of men and 27 per cent of women weigh more than 110 per cent of acceptable weight.[8] A minority of these people, of course, are very obese with body mass indices of over thirty (about 6 to 8 per cent of the population), whereas the majority fall into the mildly to moderately obese categories (body mass index twenty-five to thirty).

THE HEALTH RISKS OF BEING OBESE

The results of very many research studies, carried out both in the United States and in several European countries, now suggest that to be obese carries some risk to health.

One part of the problem of carrying too much additional weight relates directly to being overweight in itself. Hence heavy people are more prone to troubles with knee and ankle joints and, according to some authorities, with hip joints, than lightweight people. More obese women than normal-weight women develop complications in pregnancy such as toxaemia, high blood pressure, or endure a longer labour.[9]

A second aspect of being obese relates to longevity. In general, the results of several large research studies in the United States have suggested that obese people tend to die sooner than average weight people and that the likelihood of this is greater the more overweight they are.[10] The increase in mortality is steeper in people who have been overweight for longer and for people under the age of 50.[11] With extreme overweight, the extra mortality is largely accounted for by death from coronary heart disease, diabetes mellitus, digestive disease (particularly gallbladder disease), and cancer.

Of course, not everyone who contracts a serious disease or who suffers from a chronic health problem necessarily dies any earlier than a person who is fit until the very end. A third aspect of being

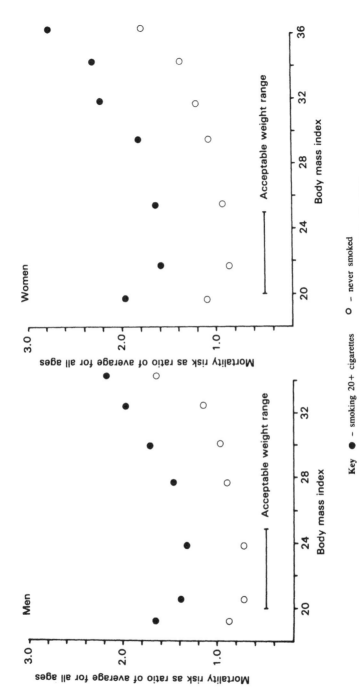

Source: Journal of the Royal College of Physicians of London Vol. 17, 1983

Figure 2 Body weight, smoking and death rates for men and women

seriously overweight therefore relates to the likelihood of becoming ill, or of developing a health problem such as high blood pressure, which is seen as being a so-called 'risk-factor' for a life-threatening illness (in this case coronary heart disease). Fat people are more prone than thin people to developing glucose intolerance, which predisposes to diabetes. There is also very substantial evidence of a strong relationship between high blood pressure and obesity.[12] Increases in body weight are also associated with increased concentrations of glucose and cholesterol in the blood, both of which predispose to greater risk of coronary heart disease.[13]

Some people would have us believe that the researchers have got it wrong: that those people who tell us that we risk our lives if we weigh more than average are merely distorting the figures to prove an ingrained prejudice against fat people. First, it is true that not all overweight people develop high blood pressure, diabetes, heart disease, or cancer. Second, it is difficult to separate out the effects of weight *per se* from the effects of eating a western diet, high in fat and low in fibre, and of taking little exercise.

Finally, it has sometimes been suggested that extreme thinness carries as much risk as obesity. This may be in part because more thin people than fat people tend to be smokers, and smoking is itself a risk factor for disease, including coronary heart disease.[14] In fact one American study which separates out the risks associated with obesity and with smoking suggests that throughout the weight range, people who smoke twenty or more cigarettes a day have double the risk of non-smokers[15] (see Figure 2). In other words, it is less dangerous to be an overweight non-smoker than a smoker of normal weight.

It is true that some overweight and obese people feel healthy and fit and live to a ripe old age. It is also true that smoking is probably more dangerous to your health than carrying extra weight. However, none of this negates the fact that, on balance, to be grossly obese stacks the odds against enjoying a long and healthy life.

Where does the risk begin?

If we accept that to be grossly obese is dangerous, the question that follows for many of us is: is being overweight or mildly obese any less dangerous, indeed should we worry about it at all?

We can define 'overweight' as having a Body Mass Index of

between 25 and 30. Let us take the example of a woman who is 5 feet 4 inches tall (1.64 metres) and weighs 11 stones and 12 pounds (75 kilograms) and who therefore has a Body Mass Index of 28.[16] There is a case for saying that to be mildly overweight is of some importance if only because the risks begin to increase with even a small increase in weight above the upper limits of the range considered to be ideal in relation to the Metropolitan Life Insurance tables. However, it would clearly be unreasonable for doctors and other health workers to insist that anyone weighing just over the 'acceptable' range of BMI 20–25 should immediately go on a diet.

An alternative strategy would be to assess the risks for each individual. Thus if the woman in the example given above were also a smoker, the line of first attack would be to suggest that she give up smoking, for even if she were to gain some weight in the process, her risk would still be very much reduced. The person's current level of fitness and whether they already had health problems such as high blood pressure, or high levels of cholesterol, would have to be taken into account. Also, the risk of developing certain diseases is raised if there is a family history. A report of the Royal College of Physicians of London in 1983 tended to follow this line, saying: 'Weight gain is particularly unwise in those with a personal or family history of coronary artery disease, hypertension or diabetes, and there is clear evidence of benefit if weight is reduced.'[17]

THE HEALTH BENEFITS OF LOSING WEIGHT

What, then, are the benefits of losing weight? One of the big questions that arises when considering the risks of being overweight or obese is whether losing weight reverses these risks. Weight loss can lead to significant reductions in both blood pressure and cholesterol levels.[18] More significantly perhaps for most people, evidence from the American life insurance companies suggests that when overweight and obese people lose weight in order to qualify for standard rates of insurance, their mortality risk returns to a normal level. In addition there are the obvious advantages: increased ability to take exercise, in itself vital for maintaining health, increased self-esteem, and all the emotional and psychological advantages of reducing one's level of disability compared with other people.

THE SOCIAL AND EMOTIONAL RISKS OF BEING OBESE

The word 'disability' in this context may surprise, or at least worry, some people. After all, given that excess weight is carried by about 30 per cent of the population, it is unusual to perceive it as a sign of physical handicap, at least until sufferers are severely restricted in some aspect of their lives. Psychologically and socially, however, there is no doubt that any degree of fatness carries with it all the pain, and the stigma, of major disability.

Whatever one's physical health status, the social and emotional aspects of being obese are usually those which have most personal impact. Fat people are often perceived as being jolly, and entirely without a care in relation to their weight. Neither in my work nor in my personal life, however, have I ever met a fat person who truly fits this stereotype. There are of course overweight people who are extremely happy, and who have an excellent sense of humour; but many feel uncomfortable about going out, particularly in situations where they might have to expose their bodies to the public gaze – communal changing rooms, swimming pools, beaches. Others avoid eating in public, imagining the disapproval of onlookers.

Attitudes to obese people

Overweight people commonly see themselves as physically unattractive or undesirable, and this clearly reflects the view that other people have of them. In many studies with children, a group renowned for saying just what they think, pictures of fat children have been rated as less likeable than those of other children.[19] For example, groups of schoolboys and girls aged 10 and 11 from different social and cultural backgrounds all over the United States were shown pictures of six children and asked to say which child they would find most easy to like. The picture they had chosen was then removed, and they were asked to make the same choice again, and so on, until all the pictures had been removed. The pictures showed: a normal-looking child, a child with crutches and a brace on its left leg, a child in a wheelchair with a blanket over its legs, a child with its left hand missing, a child with a facial disfigurement, and an obese child. In all cases, whatever the sex, education level, or social background of the children in the experiment, the picture of the obese child was liked least.[20] Pictures of fat children evoke descriptions such as 'cheats', 'sloppy', 'naughty', 'stupid', 'dirty', even at an early age.[21]

Ideas and attitudes do not just appear of their own accord, and one American researcher known for her prolific work in the obesity field, Susan Wooley, has suggested that this prejudice is somehow learned from parents at an early age. Children can learn as much from looks and actions, the most subtle nuance, often without a single word being said, as they do from direct teaching. Professor Wooley based her idea on the discovery that many parents themselves feel embarrassed about having a fat child. On one occasion, she and her colleagues were looking for photographs of obese and lean children for a research study and they spent three days in amusement parks and zoos, asking parents for permission to photograph their child. In her own words: 'No parent of a lean child ever refused; no parent of an overweight child ever agreed.'[22]

Adults do not openly express negative attitudes in the way that children do, but they are in fact just as prejudiced as children against fat people. In a replication of the experiment described above, adults were shown photographs of different children with the same result: the picture of the obese child was least liked.[23]

Obese people are at a disadvantage at work too. They are less likely to be employed, and less likely to be promoted than their thin counterparts. It has even been suggested, although there is some dispute about how far it is true, that obese executives may earn less than thin ones. There is no difference in intelligence level between thin people and fat people, but despite this, one research study found that students were less likely to be accepted for college if they were obese.[24]

Prejudice against obese patients exists among health professionals too, even in people who treat them. Thus obese patients are more likely to be perceived as being in need of psychological help than patients of normal weight and as having brought their problems on themselves.[25] This attitude was clearly reflected in a conversation I had recently with a dietitian. I had just given a lecture on the psychology of obesity, in which I had taken great pains to explain the evidence which shows that there are no differences in personality between thin people and fat people; and that while some people are more prone to putting on weight than others, they do not all eat more, so that people who cannot diet easily are not necessarily abnormal in any way. A dietitian asked: what did I think was lacking in fat people to make them continue to overeat? I explained again the point that fatter people do not necessarily overeat. In reply she said that clearly there is something psychologically 'wrong' with a fat person, that indeed there must be for the person to have 'allowed themselves to get so fat'! Sadly, it was impossible to convey to her the circularity of her argument.

Being overweight or obese puts us at a clear disadvantage, physically, socially, and emotionally, *vis-à-vis* other, slimmer people. The more overweight a person is, the greater the disadvantages. The point at which the individual decides whether he or she is overweight and needs to diet, however, varies greatly between people and depends on many factors. First, there is the vexed question of how safe it is to be overweight and when the risks of being overweight begin to outweigh (literally) the difficulties of conscious dieting. A second question revolves around the extent to which people are prepared to tolerate weighing more than the average person.

This last question is largely a social and cultural issue. Obesity takes on a different meaning from one society to another both across the world and through history. In the underdeveloped countries of the world, obesity is rare, especially in poor communities. In this context to be obese is a sign of relative wealth, and hence something to be proud of. As such, it is recognized as a sign of fertility, strength, and prosperity.[26] In some cultures, therefore, not only is it acceptable to be obese, but fatness is even a sign of beauty. The position in the western world is reversed. Obesity is now far more prevalent in people with lower socio-economic status than in the upper social classes, and this is particularly true where women are concerned. One reason for this may be financial – the cheapest foods are often those highest in fats and carbohydrates – but another possible reason is to do with attitudes towards obese people. Given that discrimination against obese people exists, in education, in employment, the climb up the social and employment ladder is likely to be more difficult, and to present more obstacles, than it does for people of normal weight.

The pressure to be slim

Negative attitudes towards the obese appear to be particularly strong in relation to women. Historically, there have been times when a healthy appetite and a large frame were to be admired, and it was considered attractive for a woman to be plump. You have only to look at the paintings of the Renaissance to see that the curvaceous woman was idealized. During this century, however, the image of womanhood has become more sylph-like. The pressure for people to be slim, and for women in particular, is reflected everywhere in the media and appears to have increased in the last twenty-five years or so.

For example, some American researchers have studied the pictures of *Playboy* magazine centre-page girls and of the winners of the 'Miss America' pageant from 1959 to 1979 and found that the ideal shapes for women have become increasingly thinner over the years. Meanwhile, the proportion of space given to material about diet and slimming in six major women's magazines increased significantly during the ten years between 1969 and 1979 compared with the previous ten years. Yet during this same period, the average weight of women under 30 was consistently several pounds heavier in 1979 than in 1959.[27] In magazines, women in a variety of states of dress and undress feature strongly in advertisements for a myriad of commodities: from chocolates, to holidays in the sun, underwear, and diet foods. All are slim. In television advertising too, the mother who uses the gentlest washing-up liquid or buys the most effective soap-powder, the girlfriend who adorns her boyfriend's new car, the woman who accepts a box of chocolates, all are slim. The fat person on the other hand is more often portrayed as stupid, a figure of fun, someone not to be taken seriously. A survey of body types portrayed on television in 1978 bears out this unrealistic representation of everyday people.[28] Fewer than 2 per cent of the actors were obese; and youth, the female sex, and positive personality attributes were all related to thinness.

Some writers have suggested that western woman is being forced to sacrifice her feminine characteristics in a struggle to fulfil an increasingly difficult role in society – as wife, as mother, as lover, and as full-time careerist in equal competition with men. Whatever the explanation, however, the pressures on women to be slim are all around us, and there can be no doubt that women are all too painfully aware of them. Women, far more than men, talk incessantly about diet, and the subject of diet is prominent in their thoughts. Only last week I was involved in a conversation which illustrates this point. I went to a meeting in a day centre for the elderly.[29] I had been asked to go in order to meet with Rosa to discuss some problems she was having with her elderly mother-in-law, a client at the day centre. When I arrived, Rosa was already there, and sitting with her was a community psychiatric nurse. I had expected to meet only with Rosa and a member of staff from the day centre and was surprised to see the nurse as well. Rosa, whom I had met a year previously, did not appear to respond to my smile of recognition; I assumed that I was mistaken and that perhaps we had not met after all, and said nothing. We were introduced, and I said, 'Hallo, I thought we had met, but I wasn't sure.' She replied, slightly embarrassed, 'Oh, I've put on some weight since last year.' The nurse pulled at an imaginary roll of fat around her own waistline and said, 'Now that spring is here, everyone is talking about diet and slimming', and as if to illustrate the point, refused a biscuit as the staff member passed the tin together with a cup of coffee. At that point another woman came in, a local general practitioner whom I had not seen for some time. 'Oh, hallo Annette,' I said, 'I didn't expect to see you here, how are you?' I turned to Rosa, sensing that she might feel intimidated by the increasing number of people in the room, and added, 'I didn't know we were having such a large meeting, did you?' Annette turned on me, and laughed. 'Large? How dare you? I'll have you know I've been on a diet and lost half a stone.'

Many people then are overweight. However, the pressure to be slim exists in some form for all of us. It is felt only too keenly by women, and probably more so for cosmetic or social reasons, than for health ones. It is perhaps not surprising that, whereas most men diet 'for health reasons',[30] women diet more often for the sake of their looks or to fit into fashionable clothes.[31]

It is easy to forget that to be conscious of 'diet' does not just mean to cut out certain items of food in order to lose weight. The kind of food we eat can also affect our health in other ways. For example, some of us are allergic to certain foods; eating a diet which has an excessive proportion of fat, or of sugar, may be harmful to us in the long term. The question 'why diet?' relates not only to whether we should aspire to be a certain shape in order to fit in with society, but also to the question of physical well-being and survival. To most people, however, the word 'diet' denotes 'slimming' and for all too many the need to lose weight is of paramount importance.

Chapter Three

CAUSES OF OBESITY

The reasons why some people are fatter than others are as varied as reasons for dieting. Some people blame the obese for having brought their problems upon themselves. Slimmers often support this idea, believing that their weight gain was caused by taking less regular exercise, by eating more than previously, or by getting married and having children. Others, dejected after countless diet attempts, claim that they must be obese because of their 'glands' or because of their 'make-up' which destines them to gain weight even if they have managed to lose it previously.

These various ideas are reflected in the endeavours of the scientists. In the words of British researchers Michael Stock and Nancy Rothwell,

> The major problems encountered by scientists and clinicians
> researching [into obesity] have been to determine whether
> excess fat accumulation is due to a high level of food intake,
> a low expenditure, or both, and to identify the underlying
> psychological, physiological and biochemical causes of the
> imbalance.[1]

One of the chief enigmas of obesity is the question of why it is that some people appear to be able to eat so much without gaining weight while others, often eating the same or less, appear to gain weight easily. There are many people who will say that they only need to look at food to gain weight. There are others who appear never to stop eating, who never gain weight, and who acquire nicknames like 'hollow-legs' from their envious friends.

In very rare cases, it is possible to become obese as a result of a serious disease affecting the part of the brain that regulates appetite. However, this is extremely unusual, and anyone suffering from such a disease would have several other symptoms far more worrying than the weight gain. Another statement often put forward by people to explain obesity in a friend or relative is that they must have a problem with their glands or their hormones. Some endocrine disorders are likely to be associated with obesity, and people who have an underactive thyroid gland may become overweight. However, these too are extremely rare causes of obesity, even in a specialist obesity clinic where people with the most serious and long-standing problems are likely to attend. What is more, there is no evidence that thyroid function is any different in obese people in general than it is in normal-weight people.[2]

FRAME SIZE

Some people place the blame for a weight problem on their frame size. 'I've got big bones', they say, making the assumption that a large frame is inevitably coupled with obesity. In general both overweight and obese people have a larger body frame size and larger musculature than lean individuals of the same height and age, and this might mean that people with larger frame size and muscle mass are also at greater risk of becoming obese; but obesity when it develops in childhood could on the other hand itself result in an increase in frame size during growth, so that the relationship between having a big frame and being obese is by no means clear.[3]

'IT'S IN MY GENES'

Another possible cause of obesity is that it may be passed on through families by genetic factors. One way in which it may be transmitted is through a single recognizable gene. This, however, occurs only in certain rare diseases, all of which have other characteristic features such as a particular facial expression, a degree of associated learning disability, or lack of muscle tone. In most people, if indeed obesity is passed on at all, it is more likely to be through genetic factors which create a predisposition to weight gain or being obese than through a biochemically traceable link.

A great deal of research energy has gone into trying to determine how far obesity can be explained by genetic factors, and how far by environmental, social ones. To a large extent, fatness level in families appears to follow family line. The probability that a parent or child will be obese is directly related to how fat the remaining family members are.[4] Thin parents rarely produce fat children. The fatter the parents are, however, the more likely it is in general that the children will be fat. Also, a child who has two fat parents has a higher chance of being fat than a child with only one fat parent. One very feasible explanation for these links is that fat people eat more than thin people and it follows that the children of fat parents will have become used to eating more so that they too become fat. There is certainly some other evidence in favour of this explanation. It is often said, for example, that husband and wife pairs grow to resemble each other. If genetic predisposition were the only cause of obesity we could not expect unrelated people who live together to grow alike in terms of fatness; but according to an American professor of anthropology and nutrition, Stanley Garn, this is exactly what happens. Spouses resemble each other in degree of fatness and go up and down in fatness level together.[5] One possibility is that they grow to be alike as a result of eating habits over the years, but it may be that fat people choose fat mates in the first place.

One way of tackling the question of genetic predisposition is to find out what happens to identical twins when they are brought up apart, in different families. If their environment were the most important influence on weight, we would expect the twins living apart to be very different. However, the weights and fatness levels of identical twins are much more similar than those of non-identical twins, whether the identical twins live together or not.

Another way of investigating genetic predisposition is to see what happens to children who are adopted. Several studies which have been able to trace adoptees and their real parents have found that there is a strong relationship between the weights of adoptees and their real parents.

So, it is likely that some of us have a stronger predisposition to becoming fat than others; but fatness is not inevitable. Unrelated people can and do grow alike in terms of fatness. There is even a significant relationship between the degree of fatness in British adults and their pet dogs![6] In other words it seems that given the right conditions almost any person or animal can grow fat.

FAT CELLS

Energy is stored in our bodies by fat. We all have a certain amount of fat, in our bodies however slim we may be. About 14–20 per cent of the adult male is fat, while for females, at 21–27 per cent, the proportion is higher. The amount of adipose tissue, or fat, in our bodies is determined by the number of fat cells and the average weight of these fat cells. Experiments with rats have shown that if infant rats are underfed, the number of fat cells in their bodies is decreased, whereas if they are overfed, their fat cells are increased permanently. It has been suggested that in children too, it is possible to establish a pattern of obesity by overfeeding in infancy, thus increasing the number of fat cells; but not all people who become obese at an early age have a large number of fat cells and some people who become fat in later life can also have larger than normal numbers of fat cells.[7] Besides, mothers will be relieved to know that there is no relationship between level of fatness in babies and young children with fatness in later life; so giving babies too much to eat does not necessarily result in obesity in adulthood, although it might in some cases. What does seem important, however, is that in some obese people who gain weight, the number of fat cells is increased; with weight loss the fat cells become smaller, but they do not seem to reduce in numbers. This could mean that once an obese person has lost weight, the fat cells are just sitting there, waiting to be filled up again, making maintenance of the weight loss particularly difficult.

ENERGY BALANCE

We maintain our weight through the balance of energy coming in in the form of food and drink, and energy being used up. Consider the analogy with a bank account. If you spend freely but do not put any money into the account, the amount of money in the bank dwindles away. If on the other hand you put money into the bank at the end of every month and spend only half what you put in, the balance grows fat and healthy. The only way to keep a consistent amount in the bank is to maintain a balance between what goes in (however much) and what comes out. In the same way, if our bodies use up more energy than we put in, we lose weight; if we put in more energy than we are able to use, we move into credit, and gain weight. In other words, we become obese when energy input exceeds energy output.

How energy is stored

Our bodies are composed of a mixture of fat, a fat-free mass or lean tissue, and a glycogen store. The fat or adipose tissue consists mainly of fat and a little water. The lean tissue is made up of protein, minerals, and about 73 per cent water.[8] Glycogen is a temporary carbohydrate energy store held mainly in liver and muscle by a large amount of water.

When we stop eating, our gut empties, the glycogen stores get used up, and the water normally bound to the glycogen is lost. This explains the very large losses people sometimes have when they first go on a starvation diet or cut out all carbohydrates. When we eat normally again, the gut contents and the glycogen store together with its associated water are replaced. This causes a rapid initial increase in weight followed by a slower rate of gain as the protein and/or fat content of the body is restored.

Metabolic rate

One of the ways in which we use energy is through our basal metabolic rate. This is the rate at which the body uses up energy when we are at rest. This is roughly proportional to the surface area of the body, so that taller people have higher metabolic rates than shorter people. Metabolic rate is also slightly higher on average in fat people than in lean people of similar height, as a proportion of the excess weight stored is lean tissue. It follows that when we gain weight, our metabolic rate goes up. This means that we are able to use up excess energy, or food, more efficiently, so that when we are fatter we can eat more without gaining increasing amounts of weight than we could previously. This contradicts the belief held by many people that fatter people have lower metabolic rates than normal. It follows, however, that when weight is lost, metabolic rate goes down. When metabolic rate drops, we need to eat less to maintain energy balance than we did before we lost the weight. Many people when they have stopped dieting breathe a sigh of relief and go back to their old ways of eating, and this is one reason why many regain their lost weight.

Thermogenesis

The second way in which we expend energy is through something called 'thermogenesis'. This is the energy used up by the body in carrying out functions other than exercise. The chief of these is dietary-induced thermogenesis, or the energy used up in processing and storing food. After we have eaten, our metabolic rate goes up temporarily and then returns to normal. There are some people who, however much they eat, never seem to gain weight, and it has been suggested that one reason why obese people gain weight so much more easily is because of a defect in the way in which energy is burned after eating. However, this idea is fairly controversial, and as yet it has not been possible to prove it either way.

Exercise

The third way in which we expend energy is through exercise. Several researchers have noted that obese people expend less energy than normal-weight people. For example, they note that lean children spend more time running about, and often eat more than obese children; that obese girls join in strenuous sports less often than thin girls, and spend less time actually moving when they do play.[9] Some have suggested that obese adults, and women in particular, spend more time in sedentary activities; others have noted that obese adults are less likely to use the stairs when an escalator is available than lean adults.[10] However, it takes more energy for a fat person to move him or herself up a flight of stairs or walk a mile than it does for a thin person, so the question of whether obese people expend less energy even if they do move around less than thin people is still in doubt. Besides, even if it were true that fat people take less exercise than thin people, this would not necessarily prove that fat people grow fat through lack of exercise, as what we are seeing may be chiefly the result rather than the cause of obesity, and there are also many lean people who take no exercise. It may also be worth noting here a point made by a British consultant in nutrition, John Garrow, that for most of us who have sedentary occupations, two hours' gentle exercise per day is about the most we can manage. At an expenditure of 5 calories per minute instead of the 1.3 calories he might expend when sitting at home, a man who goes jogging for two hours will have used about 400 calories extra.[11]

calories extra.[11] Even this amount of exercise may seem excessive to those of us who feel a glow of pride every time we shun the lift to climb one flight of stairs. Therefore for most of us the effect of exercise on energy balance may in fact be marginal. Nevertheless exercise does have beneficial effects on fitness and may be of some help in ensuring that people are able to maintain weight losses, as will be discussed in Chapter 5.

DO FAT PEOPLE EAT MORE?

So, obese people do not necessarily take less exercise than thin people, but they do have higher metabolic rates; this implies that in order to gain weight or to maintain a higher weight than slim people, they must be eating more. It is very difficult, however, to prove either that this is the case or that obese people eat more in general than people of normal weight. For one thing, we know that there are large individual variations in the amount of food eaten by people in the same age, height, and weight categories. In other words, two women of exactly the same height and age, and who weigh the same and take the same size in clothes, may eat very different amounts of food. The whole issue of whether fat people eat more than thin people is also complicated by the idea of a 'dynamic' phase as compared to a 'static' phase of obesity. There may be a period of time during which a person becomes fat through overeating, but then reduces the amount they are eating and maintains the new weight on an apparently 'normal' food intake.

One obvious way of finding out whether fatter people eat more than thinner people is to ask them. In one study 6,000 adults were asked in a twenty-minute interview to record what they had eaten in the past twenty-four hours. They were also medically examined in order to find out their heights and weights and degree of overweight. There was no evidence from the interviews that the fatter people were eating any more than the slimmer people.[12] Of course there is a major problem with asking people to record information of this nature. In the first place, merely writing down what one eats can make one self-conscious and eat less as a consequence. Second, many of us are not very good at remembering what we have eaten, unless we write it down there and then. Third, people might not be very accurate, partly because they are not very good at measuring portion sizes, and partly perhaps because they do not like to appear greedy especially if they are aware of being overweight. Still, the assumption that fat people eat more than thin people is a very powerful one, and much research time and effort has gone into investigating it. One idea that caught the interest of the researchers for a considerable period of time was that fat people eat more than thin people because of the way in which they eat. It was suggested that they eat faster than thin people, they take bigger bites, spend less time chewing in between bites, and leave less food on their plates. The evidence collected to support this idea could not of course come merely from asking people, but had to come from watching people under various conditions.

The task of observing what people eat creates just as many problems as asking them how much they eat, because understandably it is difficult to set up a situation in which one can watch people unobtrusively or in such a way as to keep from them the purpose of the observation.

Imagine the following scenario. You are an undergraduate student, and some friends have asked you to take part in an experiment about how people perceive taste. You are also somewhat overweight. The experimenter takes you to a room in which there is a large mirror, and leaves you alone with three tubs of different flavoured ice-cream, suggesting that you eat as much as you like so that you can decide which you prefer. You do not know that the mirror is in fact a two-way mirror and that the amount you 'taste' is being observed from the other side of the wall, but still the situation might seem a little less than normal. Several 'laboratory' experiments of this kind have been carried out in an attempt to find out whether fatter people eat more than thinner people, and under what conditions, with varying results. Some American researchers who themselves have carried out a great deal of work in this area, Judith Rodin and Lynn Spitzer, have concluded that of twenty-nine experiments where the purpose was hidden from the people involved, only nine showed that fat people ate more than thin people.[13]

Another way in which researchers have tried to find out whether fat people eat more than or differently from thin people is to watch what happens when people eat in restaurants. In some experiments this has meant making sure that all portions on display in a self-service restaurant are of measured quantities, and when people return their plates to the tray collection area, someone behind the racks makes an estimate of how much food is left on them. Alternatively, the experimenter might be dressed in the same uniform as the restaurant staff and might stand by the cash desk making a note of how much food and how many calories each person has helped themselves to and also of how much each person appears to weigh.

The results of experiments like these have varied. In some experiments it looks as though fatter people eat more than thinner people and in some it looks as though they eat less. Overall, however, the results suggest that there is not much difference between the amounts they eat in public. What does come out of this research, however, is that fatter people tend to eat more when the food is more palatable, or particularly tasty, than thinner people. This does not necessarily mean that fat people are more interested in tasty or sweet things than thin people, for if the most tempting desserts on a self-service counter are placed just out of reach, the thin people will work just as hard to lean over and reach them! It might simply mean that when a fatter person is eating something particularly tasty, he or she finds it more difficult to stop under some circumstances than a thin person. We will consider this possibility in more detail at a later stage, in a discussion about hunger and what makes us stop and start to eat.

One group of researchers suggested that fatter people were more likely to frequent certain restaurants. They set themselves up to observe what happened in three restaurants where there was a choice between serving yourself as much as you like on some nights, and waitress service on others. They noticed that more food overall was eaten on the self-service nights than on the waitress-service nights, but also that there was a higher percentage of obese people present on these nights than on the waitress-service nights.[14]

There are two major problems with these types of observation. In the first place, the experimenters themselves may have been biased about what they could expect to find. They were usually trained to make a rough visual estimate of how overweight a person was, but it is possible that if they expected to see more overweight people in certain settings then they would define more people as overweight in those settings and thus come up with a result that suggested that fat people are more likely to eat in those places. Second, if the findings are true, and fatter people are indeed more likely to go to restaurants where they can eat larger amounts of more fattening food, this does not necessarily mean that all fat

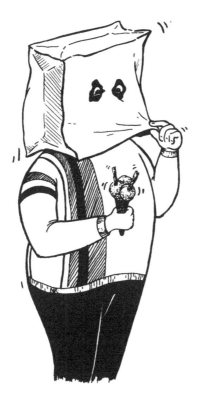

people eat more than all thin people. It may mean one of several things. People who are overweight are often very self-conscious, and reticent about being seen in public, especially in a situation where they may have to eat. Many will claim to avoid eating in public for fear that other people will say to themselves, '*She/he* shouldn't be eating that'. In one research study, in fact, observers noted that while thin people tended to eat high-calorie goodies when in company with friends, obese people did the opposite. They chose items of higher calorific value when eating alone than when eating with other people. Therefore the fatter people who do choose to eat freely in public may be a select few, who feel brave enough to defy the imagined comments of others. On the other hand they might be people who normally are dieting very hard, but who go out to eat in order to 'treat' themselves and are in fact excruciatingly hungry after long weeks on a diet!

Because eating in a restaurant in public is to some extent a very false situation (how many of us can afford to go out for lunch or dinner even once a week?), some researchers have tried to assess whether or not fat people eat more than thin people by looking at the foods they buy in the supermarket or by actually going to their homes and estimating the number of calories sitting in their larders! One survey of nearly 600 shoppers in two supermarkets in Jefferson City, USA, suggested that overweight shoppers bought food with a total calorific value greater than that bought by slim shoppers in the same shops; and that a greater percentage of the calories in the food bought by them came from fat at the expense of carbohydrate.[15] We cannot of course conclude from this that obese people eat more calories or greater amounts of fat than thin people, as people do not necessarily cook and eat everything they buy. In relation to the amount of food people keep in their larders, there appears to be a great deal of variability. It has been suggested that fatter people store more things in the high-sugar, high-calorie group of foods, such as cakes, chocolates, high-calorie condiments, than thin people, but individuals vary so greatly in their style of housekeeping that in order to draw any really firm conclusions we would have to survey every larder for miles around!

So, it is difficult to prove that fat people eat any more than thin people or that they eat faster, take bigger bites, or leave less food on their plates than thin people. Perhaps some do eat in this way, and this may be true of people who are gaining weight, and perhaps some people do go out and buy vast amounts of food and keep their larders stuffed with high-calorie, high-sugar, high-fat goodies; but people are very individual in the way that they buy, store, and consume food, and still no one has been able to prove that fat people in general eat any more than thin people.

OBESE PEOPLE WHO OVEREAT

Nevertheless, there are some fat people who do admit to eating very large amounts of food, more than they feel is reasonable. Some 50 per cent of obese people in different surveys have admitted to eating more than they need while on their diet, at least once a week, and sometimes even more often. Eating in this context feels out of control, in that people feel that they are unable to stop even though they would like to. Many people feel extremely guilty about eating in this way, and consistently vow never to do it again, to little avail.

The problem with talking about 'binge eating' is that every person's definition of a binge is different. Because the word is so loosely and subjectively used, it can mean anything from half a packet of peanuts to several extra meals, or five packets of biscuits, a whole cake, a packet of cereal, and a bowl of custard eaten one after the other. Moreover, eating in this way is not confined to obese people. Defined as eating a great deal of food, even if we are not hungry, binge eating is something that we all do from time to time. Certainly in various surveys among students, some 30–40 per cent usually admit to binge eating as often as two or three times a month or more. Binge eating appears to be something of a woman's problem in that it is reported mostly by women, and it is women who worry about it and occasionally develop more severe problems warranting medical or psychological intervention. However, there are certainly also some men who admit to having at least the occasional eating binge, so that women cannot regard the problem necessarily as entirely their own.

There was a time when it was assumed that all fat people overeat. Now we are aware that everyone overeats from time to time. Possibly some of us are rather better at using up excess fuel so that it is not easy for us to become fat. Alternatively, some of us perhaps are better at cutting down what we eat for a few days after a bout of overeating so that the extra fuel gets used up. The problem for the person who becomes obese is that presumably none of these things happens to compensate for the overeating and he or she gains weight.

THE PSYCHOLOGY OF OBESE PEOPLE

If obesity is caused by overeating then naturally the cure as far as most people are concerned is simply to stop eating. It is difficult, especially for a naturally slim person, to understand why fat people are not able to help themselves simply by going on a diet and hence losing the weight once and for all. The corollary of this is to believe, as did the dietitian I described in Chapter 2, that there must be something psychologically amiss with fat people for them to behave the way they do, to overeat (if indeed they do) and not to diet strictly and consistently.

41

Obesity and personality

As we have already seen, the fat person is often prone to being stereotyped in one way or another. One recognizable stereotype is that of the jolly fat person, always good for a laugh, often at him or herself. It has in fact been suggested that some groups of fat people are less depressed or anxious than people of normal weight; but at the same time there are many other fat people who worry a great deal or are depressed. The problem is with deciding what comes first: being depressed or anxious, or being overweight and eating more as a consequence. It is feasible that for some people being fat is a sign of underlying depression, particularly if they are people who have a tendency to overeat when depressed rather than stop eating as do other people. On the other hand, being overweight for a considerable length of time is in itself great cause for worry. Apart from the misery of having to carry extra weight, being unable to move freely, or to buy smart clothes, there is all the added pain of being discriminated against socially and occupationally, and the continual frustration inherent in failing to diet effectively. The kind of stress which results from these problems may in effect be very similar to that caused by having any chronic medical condition for which there is seldom a permanent cure; for example arthritis, or a chronic recurring bowel disorder. Often people who have these kinds of conditions suffer a higher level of overall stress or distress than other people as a consequence of having a long-standing health problem for which they have been unable to find a perfect solution.

Many people have attempted to define the obese 'personality'. To this end, countless obese people have been given paper and pencil tests, but no one has been able to prove that the personality of the fat person is any different from that of the thin person.

Psychosomatic theory

One way of looking at the causes of obesity is to make the assumption that it is a symptom of emotional conflict, and has a special meaning to the person who experiences that conflict. For example it may be an expression of hostility or anger towards other people, parents in particular; it may be a means of getting affection from other people, or it might, as many people have suggested, be a means of self-punishment. The problem with this kind of theory is that, while there are always one or two people who could fit in with each particular interpretation, it is rarely possible to find any concrete and convincing evidence for it. Another way of looking at obesity in relation to a person's life history is the view expressed by 'psychosomatic theory', put forward originally by an American psychiatrist, Hilde Bruch.[16] She suggested that certain people are unable to eat normally because of faulty learning in childhood. For example, a mother may have consistently misinterpreted her baby's needs, whether for food, cuddles, or anything else, often using food as a universal pacifier, so that as the child grew up, he or she was unable to interpret his or her own needs and learned to use food as something to turn to whatever the situation, be it in response to anger, stress, or sadness. There are indeed many people who eat more when feeling anxious or under personal threat of some kind. The problem with the theory, however, is that if fat people have learned to overeat because of past experience, we could expect eating to have the effect of reducing anxiety. In fact people who eat when they are anxious rarely experience any long-term relief from anxiety as a result of eating. As soon as the food has been eaten, most people feel worse, if anything, than they did before they started to eat. However, evidence from studies of animals suggests that certain aspects of our behaviour may not need rational explanation. For example, researchers have noticed that animals often eat in between bouts of courting their mates, or of fighting – in other words at times when they are in some way highly aroused. In the same way, eating may simply be something that we do when under stress, even if, as is the case where most of us are concerned, it does us little good either physically or psychologically.

There is no one clear cause of obesity, and even within individuals it may well be determined by a variety of factors. However, this does not mean that there is nothing anyone can do to avoid becoming fat or staying that way. The good news is that fatness is not inevitable. It is not carried by a single gene that ensures that everyone born into a certain family becomes fat, and there is no such thing as the fat personality type. There are, however, certain factors which are known to make it more likely for some of us to become overweight. If we can begin to work out what these are for us personally, then everyone may have a chance to do something about it.

Chapter Four

WHAT IS HUNGER? OR 'WHY CAN'T I JUST STOP EATING WHEN I WANT TO?'

Some dieters are so riddled with guilt about their supposed mis-demeanours that even when they go for help – to slimming clubs or to the professionals – they lay much of the blame for failure on their own weakness and lack of will-power as demonstrated by their inability to eat less and help themselves.

We make the assumption that obesity is caused by eating too much and that the cure, which is to eat less, is easily followed provided that we have that indefinable virtue called 'will-power'. Another assumption that goes along with this is that obese people have some kind of disturbance in the way they experience or respond to hunger: that either they get hungrier than other people or simply cannot recognize when they are hungry and when not.

One of the key ideas of feminist writers such as Susie Orbach, author of *Fat is a Feminist Issue*, is that in order to get over an eating problem, it is necessary to learn to distinguish stomach hunger, or real physiological hunger, from 'mouth' hunger, a desire for food which is psychological rather than biological.[1] In theory this is very sensible, and many people claim to be able to do it successfully with practice. However, there is a major problem with the concept of hunger: this is that no one has ever been able to identify or define exactly what hunger is and how it feels. The problem for a dieter is a little like that of the people in the story of the 'king's new clothes'. We are told that it is there for us all to feel, other people say that they experience it, and therefore we feel silly if we cannot ourselves feel exactly the same thing in the same way and under the same circumstances.

Ask any group of normal-weight people what they mean by the word 'hunger' and they will come up with a variety of explanations, but they will not all come up with the same ones. Some people will claim that their stomachs rumble, others will describe themselves as feeling empty, others as feeling hollow, some even as having pain or an ache in their stomachs. Yet some people experience none of these symptoms at all when they are hungry or when they have not eaten for several hours. The sensation of hunger does not in fact depend only on what goes on in the stomach. It is possible even for animals or people who have had the nerves serving the stomach removed to experience hunger. Other factors such as the level of sugar circulating in the blood, and messages carried in hormones, have an effect on the feeling of hunger or its opposite, satiety. The exact mechanisms by which we start to eat or stop eating are as yet not fully understood. What is increasingly clear, however, is that whatever the physiological controls on eating, these can be overridden in many ways.

An understanding of some of the ways in which our bodies can be fooled into needing more food may help us to avoid some of the temptations around us and find a way of eating less without necessarily feeling deprived.

THE EFFECT OF OUR THOUGHTS ON WHAT WE EAT

One implication of the idea that we automatically know when we have had enough to eat is that the nutritional properties of foods are recognized by our digestive systems. If this happened we would know when to stop eating without having to devise our own system of control such as counting calories or units of food. In actual fact things do not seem to work in this way, at least not in the short term, over a few hours.

The easiest way for a scientist to find out how people regulate the amount they eat is to use food which is uniform, and therefore easily measured. In one such experiment, the Americans Hashim and Van Itallie gave obese patients a uniform-tasting liquid nutrient.[2] They had to help themselves to the drink whenever they felt hungry. The experiment lasted for three weeks, and at the end of the time, all the patients had lost weight. Perhaps the people in the experiment could not tell how much they needed because they could not see what they were taking in. The results of another, more recent, experiment suggested that on the other hand we can be fooled by the appearance of what we eat into eating more or less. American psychologist

Susan Wooley conducted an experiment in which she gave sixteen obese and sixteen normal-weight students a special drink, followed by a snack meal.[3] There were two types of special drink: low calorie and high calorie. The experiment was repeated on each of four consecutive days at lunchtime and the subjects were given one of the special drinks, designed half the time to look like a rich milk shake, and half the time to look like a low-calorie drink. Whether the subjects had the low- or the high-calorie drink before their meal had no effect on how much they ate afterwards; but the appearance of the drinks did have an effect on how many sandwiches they ate. The subjects helped themselves to fewer sandwiches and said they felt fuller after the drink which looked like a high-calorie drink, than they did after the drink designed to appear low in calories. Moreover, there was no difference between the normal-weight people and the obese people in the ability to compensate for the number of calories they had already taken by eating more or less afterwards. This experiment shows us that we can make decisions to eat or not based not on internal, physiological signals, but on external things such as the appearance or the taste of what we eat.

THE INFLUENCE OF GOOD TASTE ON WHAT WE EAT

An important feature of the food dispenser experiment described on page 45 is that the food dispensed was extremely boring to eat. It may have contained all the nutrients anyone could want, but certainly none of the people using it spent more than the minimum amount of time necessary to get food out of it. The taste of what we eat is very important to us, and the better something tastes, the more we are likely to consume. Researchers have found that in general the more tasty or palatable a food is to an individual, the more of that food the person will eat. Quite normal-weight people taking part in experiments on food intake will put on weight given a situation where they are allowed to eat as much as they like of good-tasting food over a period of several days. This finding is unlikely to come as a surprise to those readers who know that on holiday in a hotel where the food is good and plentiful, they can put on weight with the greatest of ease.

'VARIETY IS THE SPICE OF LIFE'

Part of what makes food nice to eat or palatable is of course its variety. There are a few very self-controlled people who at a dinner party will decline the dessert course; but far more of us are happy to eat our way through an hors-d'oeuvre, followed by a main course with several different accompaniments, and will go on, however full, to eat a dessert or even sample several if our hosts have been extravagant enough to offer a variety! One way of looking at this would be to describe it as pure gluttony. However, variety has been found to have an effect on people in general which suggests that the explanation of gluttony is too simple.

Some experiments by Barbara Rolls and her colleagues have demonstrated the effect of variety on eating very neatly.[4] In one experiment, for example, they invited student nurses to a sandwich lunch. The nurses ate one-third more sandwiches when offered a choice of sandwiches with four different fillings than they did when offered only one filling. The people who took part in these experiments had to fill in a questionnaire about how the food tasted. Foods already eaten became less pleasant to taste, whereas other foods were rated as more pleasant, which explains why they were more readily eaten. The effect is greater the more different the foods are. Thus, eating one kind of meat reduces the pleasantness of other meats as well, but might make other foods, such as sweet foods, seem more pleasant.

It has been suggested that the effect of variety on eating may be one explanation of why people get fat. This idea comes from observing what happens to rats when they are given a variety of foods; if they are given a variety of palatable foods over a period of several weeks instead of standard 'chow', as food given to rats is usually called, they gain weight. It is always dangerous to extrapolate from animal experiments to drawing conclusions about humans; however, it seems quite feasible that confronted with a large degree of variety in the supermarket, in restaurants, and especially at the table in our homes, we may all be influenced unknowingly in the direction of eating more than we need.

HISTORICAL AND SOCIAL INFLUENCES ON WHAT WE EAT

We are reminded by food historian Stephen Mennell in his book *All Manners of Food* that a variety of tasty dishes was not always available to us as it is today.[5] Until the early part of the nineteenth century, harvest failure, and therefore famine, were part of life in Europe, and in many areas the worry about whether there would be enough to eat to avoid starving to death was very real. With the advent of the nineteenth-century increase in trade and in the reliability of food supplies, people who moved up through the social strata were confronted with unaccustomed amounts of freely available food and began to overeat and to have problems with their weight. Gastronomic writers, who previously had written about how to tempt the appetite by creating more and more palatable dishes, began to introduce the idea of moderation into their books. Another change that Mennell notes is that the contrast between festivals and other normal times in the year has become less marked. With fast worldwide distribution and new ways of preserving and storing foods, foods normally eaten only at certain times of year or during certain festivals are now available all the year round. With each new large supermarket built, there appears to be an increasing variety of foodstuffs on the shelves. This means that people can eat what they like whenever they like, and choose to eat the foods which they find most palatable whether they are really in season or not.

We often make the assumption that people have a natural ability to eat just enough to stay alive and in good health; that somehow each one of us knows just how much he or she needs and in what combination. The historical facts, however, appear to contradict this picture. In Roman times, the Emperor Augustus was so worried about the gluttony of his people that he tried to limit the amount of food bought by limiting the expenditure allowed on certain meals. When plenty has been available, gluttony, or at least overeating, appears to have been the order of the day. For example, at the court of Louis XIV of France, we are told of the 'king's prodigious consumption' and of the 'overeating of the French nobility'.[6]

WHY DO WE EAT WHAT WE DO?

Readers who are interested in healthy eating might now be saying:

'Surely most people would rather eat what is good for them than food of low nutritional value or cheap convenience food?' Sadly, the kind of food we eat is more often determined by all kinds of factors other than an inborn knowledge of what is good for us.

Much of what we learn about food comes from experience. Most of us eat what our mothers cook for us, which on the whole is fairly similar to what our neighbours or our relatives eat; and mother's cooking often tastes best. We grow to like novel foods only through experience, otherwise we tend to stick with what we are used to. Our culture tells us what foods to eat and what foods to avoid. For example, we all know that certain items must be avoided because they are poisonous. Certain foods are treated as delicacies in some cultures and avoided by others: only recently have the British considered eating the frogs' legs so beloved of the French. We learn to avoid other foods because they are vetoed by our religion (meat by some Hindus, pork by Jews and Moslems).

On the other hand, food also has meaning attached to it. Food can have social and class implications – caviare is for the rich, and there is a world of difference between the food served in the café where the long-distance driver takes his lunch-break and the food served in the restaurant of a five-star hotel in the evening. Food habits may change with the social climate, albeit not always for the better, and, like clothes, tend to follow fashions. Thus, to take an extreme example; on the island of Nauru in the Pacific, the islanders, in becoming 'westernized' in the 1960s, replaced their traditional meal pattern with one of irregular snacking of high-carbohydrate foods. As a consequence the incidence of diabetes has very much increased in comparison with that on other Pacific islands with a less westernized life-style.[7]

The way in which food likes and dislikes can be affected in a subtle way by social factors is very neatly illustrated by a series of experiments with children carried out at the University of Illinois by Leann Birch and her colleagues.[8] They talked to sixty-four 3- to 5-year-old children and found out about the kinds of snack foods they liked. They found some 'neutral' foods for each child, neutral in that the child neither particularly liked nor disliked them. Then they offered the foods to the children in several different situations. They found that if the foods were presented together with adult attention, or as rewards, the children grew to like them more than they had at the beginning of the experiment. Also, this increased liking for the previously neutral foods continued for several weeks after the end of the experiment. If, on the other hand, the foods were presented in a matter-of-fact way at normal snack times, the children's liking for them did not increase. Thus it looks as though liking for a particular food can be influenced by the kind of setting in which it is introduced.

In another experiment, a group of children were given milk shakes which they neither liked nor disliked, in one of two situations: in one situation, the children were told that if they drank their milk shakes, they would get to see a film as a reward. In the other situation, the children were given the milk shakes, and also saw the film, but there was no talk of rewards. All the children enjoyed their special 'snack' sessions, but the children who had had to drink their milk shakes in order to get their reward liked the milk shake less than they had previously, whereas the other children liked it slightly more.[9] So when parents tell their children, 'Eat up your vegetables and I'll give you . . .', they may be inadvertently decreasing their child's liking for the vegetables, and increasing their liking for the reward, often something sweet, and exactly the kind of food parents are trying to dissuade their children from eating!

Nevertheless, it is not easy to manipulate children, or adults for that matter, into preferring what is good for them to high-fat, high-sugar foods. Television advertising has a strong influence on children's preference for these foods, but similar advertising aimed at persuading children to choose high-nutrition foods such as fruits and vegetables does not appear to have nearly as powerful an effect.

'A sweet tooth'

This raises the question of why it is that sweet, sugary, and high-fat foods have such a powerful appeal to adults and children alike. To some extent, liking for sweet things appears to be inborn. Babies smile when they taste sweet things, and frown when they taste bitter. Throughout the ages and across the world, people choose to eat sugary foods when they are available and affordable.

It is not altogether clear how far having a 'sweet tooth' is inevitable for some people, and how far it can be avoided by correct handling in childhood. If sweet taste is indeed predetermined, it may, however, be modified as a result of experience. In an attempt to investigate this, researchers Beauchamp and Moran gave 140 newly born babies at Pennsylvania hospital in Philadelphia a special taste test.[10] They gave them sterile water to drink, and on another occasion they gave them water which had some sucrose, or sugar, diluted in it. Each time they measured how much of the solutions the babies had drunk. Six months later, they asked each of the babies' mothers to give them a record of what their babies had eaten and drunk over the past week. On the whole, the babies appeared to be eating the same kinds of things at six months; but one-third of the babies were having sweetened water. The researchers then repeated the taste test they had done when the babies were born. The babies who were not used to sweetened water drank less in the test relative to pure water than they had at birth; and they drank less sweetened water than the babies who were used to drinking it. So perhaps our natural liking for certain foods can be tempered by experience.

Experience can have a very powerful effect on our willingness to eat certain foods; but a question that has continued to puzzle researchers is that of why it is that some foods are so much more preferable to us than others, and so much more difficult to stop eating. One possibility is that eating foods containing sugar has a biochemical effect on the body which in effect is like addiction, leading to greater hunger for sweet, starchy foods. On the other hand it may be that simply eating what one likes whets the appetite for yet more food. This seemed to be the result of an experiment carried out by some researchers in Leeds.[11] They asked some students to check off on a list of foods what were their favourite foods, and which foods they would eat but could do without. They then gave the students lunch. To half the students they gave a lunch consisting of the foods they liked best, and to the other half they gave a lunch consisting of their less preferred foods. At intervals during the experiment the students were asked to fill in questionnaires about how hungry they were and how much they felt like eating. The students' desire to eat returned more quickly after meals in which they had eaten the food they preferred than after meals in which they had eaten the non-preferred food.

Another interesting finding suggests that the way in which nutrients are combined may have an important effect on our preference for certain foods. We rarely choose to taste sweetness, as in say a spoonful of sugar, on its own, but we do enjoy sweetened foods. In the same way, we rarely enjoy a 'fatty' or a 'creamy' taste on its own, but researchers have shown that cream is more liked if its sugar content is increased.[12] This may have some bearing on why our desire for high-fat, high-sugar foods such as chocolate and ice-cream far outweighs any possible nutritional needs we may have for these 'foods'.

The important thing to remember about all the factors that affect our appetite for various foods is that they influence fat people and thin people equally. Obese people are no less accurate at judging what they have eaten when its calorific value is disguised; and where food is plentiful and tasty, both slim people and obese people can put on weight.

Some researchers have suggested that perhaps obese people are more sensitive to sweet-tasting food than thin people in that it produces in them the desire to eat more. Others have suggested that obese people are insensitive to sweet taste, in that the feedback system which is said to tell normal-weight people when they have taken in enough food is missing or faulty. However, the evidence in support of these various ideas is inconclusive. Where differences have been found, they may well have been caused not by the difference between fat people and thin people *per se*, but by the possible difference between people who are dieting and therefore in a state of chronic mild hunger or deprivation, and people who are not on a diet.

Eyes bigger than your stomach

All around us there are sights, images, sounds, and smells that remind us of food: for example, pictures of our favourite foods leap out at us from advertisements on hoardings, on the television. At the cinema, larger than life advertisements for drinks and snack foods send small crowds of people hurrying down the aisles to queue in front of the light which marks the confectionery holder; and the rustle of snack wrappings reaches a crescendo by the time the lights go down again for the main feature. Tempting smells waft from the baker shops and the coffee houses; certain times of day remind us that it is time to eat, or to sit down with a cup of tea or coffee.

One idea that has greatly interested researchers is that fat people are more responsive to these kinds of signals or 'cues' to eat than thin people. If indeed fat people were more sensitive to the sight of food than thin people and could not help but eat whenever they saw food or were reminded of food, this would provide a very plausible explanation of why it is that some people grow fat more easily than others. This idea was first put forward by American psychologist Stanley Schachter in the 1960s.[13] He believed that normal people eat in response to internal, physiological stimuli, such as hunger contractions in the stomach; obese people on the other hand are less responsive to these kinds of signals, and respond instead to external signals associated with food. Thus, he would expect obese people to eat more readily at the sight of food than thin people, and to be less ready to eat if food is not easily available; obese people might be more inclined to eat if the clock tells them it is supper-time, or if they see other people eating. In one experiment, Schachter and his colleague altered the clocks so as to trick people into believing it was near dinner-time. He left snack crackers on the table so that the participants, students who were unaware of the purpose of the experiment, could help themselves. The obese students in the study ate almost twice as many snack crackers when they believed it was just after 6.0 pm as they did when the clock showed 5.20 pm. The normal-weight people, however, did the opposite, eating more snack crackers when they believed it was 5.20 pm than when they thought it was 6.00 pm – as if they were saving themselves for their dinners. This kind of experiment has been repeated many, many times but in fact it is not always the fatter people who respond more readily to the so-called external cues. There are indeed differences between people in the degree to which they can be tricked by things they see and hear around them into eating, but the differences do not correspond neatly with degree of overweight. In other words, people of all weights can be tempted to eat by a variety of sights, sounds, smells, and even thoughts to do with food; and, as we have seen in Chapter 3, will put on weight when food is available, plentiful, and tasty.

The chief difference which may emerge between groups of people who gain weight under these circumstances is that some are able to lose the weight again afterwards, and others are not. Therefore, while we cannot blame people who grow fat for having eyes bigger than their bellies, we perhaps have to be aware that a tendency to eat at the mere sight, smell, or thought of food can trick some of us into experiencing 'hunger' far more often than we need to. This aspect of hunger has a particularly strong impact in a world where food is all around us, easily available, enticingly packaged, and needs less and less preparation before it is ready to eat.

CONCERN ABOUT DIETING

The more food there is available, and the more we are tempted to try new products, the more concerned some of us become about our weight and about dieting. While there are some people who never worry about their weight, whose weight remains fairly stable, and who never diet, there are others, as we all know, who spend a great deal of time thinking about food and diet, who feel guilty when they think they are overeating, and whose weight may fluctuate considerably within a short period of time.

People who experience these worries have been called by the Americans Herman and Mack, 'restrained eaters'.[14] They gave a questionnaire designed to measure the restraint phenomenon to some normal-weight students and divided them up according to their scores into high- and low-restrained subjects. (In other words, there were two groups of people, one characterized by a high degree of concern about their weight and diet, and the other less concerned or not concerned at all, but all of them of normal weight.) They gave the students either a small or a large milk shake and then left them to help themselves to snack foods. The students who had scored high on the restraint scale (i.e. were concerned about their weight and diet) ate more than the low scorers and also ate more after the large milk shake than after the small one, which is exactly the opposite of what we would expect. This finding, where people concerned about dieting and weight eat more the more they have already had, has been demonstrated in many subsequent experiments. The difference in the amounts of food eaten does not reflect weight differences between the people, but appears to be associated with 'restraint' or degree of concern about weight. This interesting finding is quite similar to the tendency of some dieters to eat more the more worried they are about their weight, for example, to continue to eat large amounts the day after having a grand slap-up meal. This implies that the phenomenon may have something to do with what goes on in the minds of dieters when they feel they have overeaten, rather than something which is purely physiological. In fact, researchers have found that restrained eaters who believe what they have just eaten to be high in calories eat more afterwards than if they believe what they had eaten was low in calories. Similarly, restrained eaters led to believe they are about to be asked to eat something high in calories, such as a milk shake, rather than something low calorie such as a salad, will also eat more than unrestrained eaters. These findings have quite important implications for the would-be dieter: they suggest that just *thinking* that one has eaten too much or is about to, whether true or not, can lead to overeating.

Thinking about food and about the possibility of breaking one's diet can be very stressful for a dieter or for someone who is always watchful of his or her weight. In a sense, it appears as though these factors are the trigger to push would-be dieters temporarily to loosen their grip on their characteristic 'restraint' and overeat or even binge. Stress itself appears to have a similar effect. Many people admit to eating more when they are depressed or anxious, and in several research studies, people scoring high on the 'restraint' scale have eaten more or described themselves as eating more when depressed than 'unrestrained' eaters.

Hunger, then, is a very complex phenomenon. It comes not just from within, but is influenced by a host of external factors, and even by our very thoughts and feelings. Most of the time we may have little awareness of, and therefore little control over, these hidden influences. However, if we can begin to understand them, we may begin to appreciate why dieting is no easy undertaking. We may be able to stop blaming the failure of dieting on the personality of the dieter or on greed itself. Instead, we may begin to seek the origin of the problems in a combination of social and psychological influences which together with biological influences shape our behaviour.

Chapter Five

SUCCESSFUL SLIMMING

THE 'JOYS' OF SLIMMING

Much of the 'joy' of slimming must surely lie in a successful outcome, when it occurs. If feeling fat turns people inward, lowers self-esteem, and prevents people from holding their heads up high when they venture out, then successful slimming has the opposite effect. Successful slimmers describe themselves as altogether happier, more self-confident, more able to take part in group and physical activities than previously. Because of the unfortunate tendency of fashion designers to make acceptable-looking clothes in nothing larger than a size 12 (US 10), the women are able, perhaps for the first time in many years, to buy fashionable clothes which make them feel 'normal'. Successful losers as a group take a new pride in their appearance, are more satisfied with the way their bodies look, and are less determined to avoid looking in every shop window they pass for fear of seeing a chance reflection of themselves. Many people are able with their new-found confidence to give up unsatisfactory jobs or spouses to seek out new ones; and people who are happy with their lot seem to become more contented, basking in the heightened attention from friends and loved ones, and enjoying a more active social life.

Some of these effects are for many slimmers the *raison d'être* of dieting. The new and trim figure, the burgeoning self-confidence, the increase in assertiveness or social activity; these are the shining goals at the end of the long road of 'The Diet'.

SLIMMING AS A PASTIME

For those who have not yet reached the end, slimming does have its own intrinsic pleasures. One of these must surely be the pleasure of the enthusiast. Slimmers have their own particular kind of language and topics of conversation, and the fascination for slimmers of a good diet moan can be paralleled only by the fascination for topical stories of sailors and downhill skiers. Dieters take great interest in discussion of this diet or that diet, the success or failure of one or other friend.

Many people derive a certain pleasure from membership of a slimming club. This may be difficult to understand given that some clubs are run in such a way that members feel chastised if they do not lose weight each week. One possible reason for allowing oneself to be shamed in this way is that many people, women in particular, feel extremely guilty about the lack of self-control which they believe is demonstrated by their overweight. Many writers have drawn an analogy between slimming and religion, with its often strict laws and opportunity for obedience or sin.[1,2] In this setting, a slimming group can provide a forum for confession, and with the forgiveness of the group and the leader the wayward dieter can feel free to begin again with a clean slate. Nevertheless, the pleasure is somewhat tainted by the flavour of self-punishment, or even of masochism that is involved.

Not all slimmers of course are so obsessed by their weight and diet as to take the consequences of losing or not losing weight so seriously. For some people, a slimming club provides a place to meet just like any other club. In the western world the extended family is fast disappearing and whatever the benefits of this change the negative aspect is that people are increasingly isolated as they pick up their roots and move house to work far away from friends and relatives. Often workmates become the sole source of social contact. For a woman at home contact may be altogether missing unless she has a child of toddler group age and can meet other mothers for a while amidst the clatter of a nursery group. Otherwise, any focus for meeting other people can create for her an island of familiarity in an otherwise threatening sea of alienation and isolation. This may be one reason why the vast majority of slimming club members are women. What better than a group with a common aim, to dispel fatness, source of so much dissatisfaction and unease for so many. It is not surprising that many slimmers, even when they do not lose the desired amount of weight, are happy to continue with membership of their clubs for several weeks at a time.

PAYING FOR SUCCESS

There is another aspect of belonging to a slimming club, going to a special beauty clinic, or staying on a health farm, that cannot be ignored. This is the issue of payment. Many people believe that the more you have to pay for a service, the better it must be. We see this, for example, in some attitudes to private medicine. 'I saw the top man' is a comment that I have heard many people make about doctors they have seen. In answer to my question about how they knew he was the top man, the reply often says more about the address of his practice or the cost of the appointment than about his credentials. In addition, if we feel that we have paid heavily for a service, we are loath to admit, even to ourselves, that it has not helped us. The amount a slimmer has to pay to join a club or, in the United States, a professional slimming programme, can have a marked effect on the success of the treatment, provided of course that the treatment itself has some intrinsic therapeutic benefit. Programmes which charge very small fees are characterized by higher drop-out rates than programmes which charge higher fees; expensive programmes have lower drop-out rates and therefore may produce better losses than low-cost programmes, but they may select out only the most strongly motivated people in the first place, as fewer people are prepared to join. For every dieter there may be an optimum payment that would help to ensure commitment to a programme.

DIET LITERATURE

Not everyone is comfortable joining a club or talking to a profes-sional, and much of the information that dieters glean about dieting and how to do it comes from books and magazines. For the person struggling alone with a diet, reading a magazine with its problem pages, its recipes for low-calorie dishes, provides endless pleasure. For one thing, we all love to read about other people who suffer the same problems as we do. There is the satisfaction that there is always someone worse off than we are; and there is the vicarious fascination of reading how others have dealt with problems similar to our own. When I first set about writing this book, several people declared that they hoped I would include several case studies, as they loved to read stories about other people and their problems.

One advantage of reading diet literature then, is that at best it can be a source of emotional support. At worst, of course, it may be misguided, and in fact given the confusion that exists in the diet world about what is good for dieters and what is not, it is extremely difficult for the would-be dieter to make an informed choice of reading material. Nevertheless, reading does have some general advantages. One of these is that the written word can help us to understand instructions better than the spoken word. It may be difficult for us to understand information given to us by other people, often because they themselves are not very good at explaining. If a doctor or a dietitian gives us a diet, it helps to have it written down so that we understand which foods to eat and which to avoid, together with an explanation of why. Having something in writing also helps us to remember what to do. The finding that patients forget 50 per cent of what a doctor has told them within five minutes of a consultation is one that is often quoted. It is worth mentioning here, because it may apply equally well to any other information given to us by a professional or at a slimming club.

In the United States, there are many centres where people can go for professional help with weight reduction. Because of the large numbers of people passing through these centres, the most economical way to treat clients is often in groups, sometimes with a standard treatment package. Many centres include a self-help treatment manual as part of their package. These manuals contain week-by-week instructions about how to keep to the diet, instructions about how to monitor progress with weight and eating, and sometimes advice for trouble-shooting when problems arise.

Several researchers have investigated the possibility of using these manuals on their own, without the client having to meet the therapist at all, or at least only now and again. Some have found that people lose as much weight as a result of reading a manual as others who attend a group where they meet their therapist every week. Others have found that people do even better with a combination of reading together with meeting a therapist on a few occasions than people who see their therapist frequently. Thus some people benefit more from being left to their own devices and finding their own solutions to problems than from regular advice from another person.

Other people, however, prefer the support and encouragement they get from having someone to talk to. In one research study which compared regular group meetings with a correspondence course which covered the same material, the ten women who attended the group lost more weight and dropped out of treatment less readily than the ten women who were on the correspondence course.[3]

WHO ARE THE SUCCESSFUL SLIMMERS?

If there is a difference between people who enjoy successful slimming on their own and those who need a group to encourage them when the going gets tough, does this mean that some people are better at losing weight than others? The successful slimmer, in particular the woman who achieves the body shape craved by so many, is admired by others. She is often seen as having some special characteristic that differentiates her from the woman who cannot lose weight by dieting, the 'slob'.[4]

For many years, people have assumed that it should be possible to identify the difference between people with 'will-power', successful dieters, and people who fail to lose weight. One common belief, for example, is that if a person wants to lose weight badly enough because he or she fears the consequences of not doing so, then he or she will succeed. However, people who need to lose weight for a physical reason appear to do no better than those who want to lose weight for a psychological reason.[5] Moreover, no one has been able to identify a personality variable that distinguishes good losers from poor losers, and this line of investigation has now more or less been dropped.

There are, however, some differences between people who do well and people who fail with diets. One difference is that people who believe they will do well, who believe perhaps that they have good self-control, are the people most likely to succeed.[6] Often they are people who have not tried dieting too many times before, and therefore have not had the undermining experience of failure. Some of them are people who have tried several times already, but this time they have developed a definite plan of action. It helps too if they are people who know themselves well; who know their own shortcomings, who know just how much they can expect themselves to change, and the point at which their self-control will give way, so that perhaps they are less likely to put themselves into situations where they will be unable to keep to the diet. This may partly explain an apparent contradiction thrown up by research in this area. In some research studies, dieters who claimed to be able to avoid eating for emotional reasons were the ones who were most successful at dieting; but in other studies, including our own, the people who most freely admitted to eating for emotional reasons were the ones who did best. The tendency to overeat under stress is not necessarily a bar to successful dieting as long as the dieter recognizes the problem and is therefore half way to devising a strategy to cope with it.

So to some extent success is engendered by an attitude of mind. A would-be slimmer reading this may be saying, 'I know I'm a failure at dieting. I've got no self-control. I might as well give up now.' This is not necessarily the case. Attitudes are not fixed and unchangeable; they depend on our knowledge of the world, and so can change with experience. Yesterday's failed dieter may learn self-control through self-understanding, or self-love. She does not have to be tomorrow's 'slob'.

PREDICTING DIET SUCCESS

The people who succeed with dieting also have other important characteristics in common. The first of these is to do with the kind of support they get from people around them. An important finding of research into professional programmes is that people who enrol in a group often do better than people who see a therapist on their own. Possibly the camaraderie, the rewards which come from being encouraged by one's peers to do well, and the pressure to come into line when one slips back into old habits, are powerful agents of change. In the United States, where obesity is recognized as a problem of great national importance, some organizations have taken this idea seriously and have set up slimming groups which their staff are strongly encouraged to attend, sometimes as part of a wider programme of health education and stress avoidance at work.

The influence of family

The family is the most important social group in our lives. The role of one's immediate family is of crucial importance in the success or otherwise of slimming projects. Most slimmers know that spouses, children, parents, and even friends can be instrumental in sabotaging a diet or encouraging changed eating habits. One lady I met who needed to lose upwards of thirty pounds for the sake of her health described one of the pleasures which she and her husband shared at the end of a long day of looking after their three small children. They would watch television in bed while eating large bacon sandwiches prepared by her husband. To allow her husband to eat his bedtime 'snack' alone would have been very difficult for this lady, especially as part of the enjoyment for both of them was eating together; on the other hand, to ask him to forgo his snack too would mean asking him to break a long-established habit. In fact, because the couple got on well together, it was not too difficult for them to work out alternative ways of relaxing together or of doing things for each other. In a similar situation, many other people have faced repeated if unconscious sabotage by family members unwilling to change their old habits.

The involvement of partners has been taken very seriously in recent years and many research studies have been designed to include them in treatment. In one programme, husbands were taught the same weight loss techniques as their wives and encouraged to keep records both of their wife's eating and of their own; they were taught to reward their wives for specific 'good behaviour' (agreed beforehand) and encourage them to take part in activities which did not involve eating.[7] The wives whose husbands took an active part in their programme in this way managed to continue losing weight for longer than wives whose husbands were not directly involved.

This does not mean of course that everyone who goes on a diet needs to force their spouse to do the same. Other researchers have found that merely getting husbands' agreement to help, for example making a husband's involvement a condition of his wife's acceptance on to a programme, is enough to ensure that the women do well.

The key to all this may of course have less to do with what husbands and wives actually do to help their partners lose weight than with the way the couple gets on together. Dieting is difficult; and the difference between having a partner who can support, encourage, and praise in contrast to having a partner who criticizes, blames, and is oblivious to changes for the better, can make all the difference between success and failure.

The same factors come into play where children and slimming are concerned. The support of parents is perhaps even more important for children, as they are the main providers of food and the people who decide what kind of diet their children will live on. To take an extreme case, no one can expect a child to favour fruit, lean meat, and vegetables when the rest of the family exists on a diet of sausages, pies, and cakes. Unfortunately, the onus for helping their children to lose weight appears to have fallen chiefly on the mothers, as implied by the kinds of programme adopted in research studies. Nevertheless, children whose mothers have been taught specific skills for rewarding their child for choosing the right foods, getting involved in more activities which involve exercise, and helping them to keep to their diets in a positive, non-punishing way, have more quickly succeeded with diets than children whose parents have not been given this kind of help.

Changing life-styles

Many of the people who succeed in losing weight say that one of the key aspects of slimming and of keeping their weight down in the future is the ability to make overall changes in life-style. They learn to enjoy eating in a different way. For some people, going on a diet may have served as an introduction to high-fibre, low-sugar, and low-fat foods: they may for the first time experience the feeling of well-being associated with eating more natural foods such as vegetables and fruit, in contrast to the sluggish feeling often engendered by eating high-fat, high-sugar snack foods with little nutritional value.

Another change which appears to differentiate successful from unsuccessful slimmers is a tendency to take more exercise while they are dieting and to continue to include exercise in their daily lives.

Does taking exercise help you to lose weight?

The question of how far exercise can speed weight loss is one that has been hotly debated. We all know that in order to lose weight it is necessary to use up more energy than one takes in; so it follows that taking exercise should help to tip the scales in the desired direction. In terms of calories, however, we would need to walk several miles in order to use up the energy provided by a few squares of chocolate.

One group of researchers in San Francisco compared the effects in two groups of moderately overweight women on a metabolic ward of a low-calorie diet and a slightly higher calorie diet combined with exercise. The people in the diet-alone group had to reduce their calorie intake by 50 per cent, and the people in the diet-plus-exercise group had to reduce their intake by 25 per cent and increase their level of physical activity by 25 per cent. The people in the diet-alone group lost more weight than the diet-plus-exercise group.[8] The problem is that few people who are overweight, even if only to a moderate degree, are fit enough to take enough exercise for it to have any appreciable effect. Moreover, while people who take exercise eat less in the short term, taking a moderate amount of exercise appears to lead to an increase in food intake in most people.[9]

Nevertheless, some people have suggested that exercise can have other effects which help to speed weight loss. One of these suggestions is that exercise can prevent the decrease in metabolic rate which occurs during a restricted diet. However, there is no clear evidence from studies which accurately measure metabolic rate that this is the case.[10] Another suggestion is that exercise leads to an increased resting metabolic rate not only during the exercise itself but also during the rest of the day. If this were true it could mean that taking exercise could help us to 'burn up' energy faster throughout the day and thus lead to faster weight loss. This is a fairly controversial idea, however, and after a careful review of the evidence, John Garrow has concluded that

> exercise at a level which obese people might be able to
> tolerate has no detectable effect on metabolic rate a few
> minutes after the exercise has ceased, although there may be a
> prolonged effect on metabolic rate after more severe exercise
> continued to exhaustion in well-trained subjects.[11]

In other words, while taking vigorous exercise might lead to changes in the metabolism of lean, fit, athletic types, it is still doubtful whether it can have any appreciable effect on unfit, overweight people.

Exercise does, however, have some benefits for the dieter. One of these is that while it does not lead to an increase in lean tissue, it can help to preserve the lean tissue we already have, as a greater proportion of the weight lost with the help of exercise, compared with dieting alone, is due to fat loss. It should, however, be stressed that this probably depends on how vigorous the exercise is. Anyone who is overweight and not accustomed to exercise should take things very gradually and in any case should check with their doctor as to their fitness to take up an increased level of exercise in the first place.

Other benefits are those which would apply to anyone who engages in exercise, whether overweight or not. Taking regular exercise is said to reduce blood pressure and increase cardiovascular fitness; and it has even been suggested that it may have a protective effect against certain cancers.[12]

There is also a great deal of research evidence which suggests that there is an association between exercise and improvements in mood, especially for people who are moderately depressed or anxious. This does not necessarily mean that exercise causes happiness. It could be that the types of people who take exercise are different from the types who lead a more sedentary life. Or it could be that taking exercise helps us to distract ourselves from daily problems in just the way that relaxing or listening to music does. Certainly the sense of achievement gained from increasing our level of fitness can have an important effect on increasing self-confidence, a feeling that is vital to the would-be slimmer.

Another theory which may prove to explain the association is that exercise leads to biochemical changes in the body which can have a euphoric effect. Exercise is certainly an activity which for some people can become almost addictive in terms of the rewards it brings. Hetty Einzig, in the book *Dieting Makes You Fat*, extols the joys and virtues of exercise in a very compelling way:

> Exercise allows us to rediscover the child's joy of simply being alive. . . . I had not realised just how much time I spent looking at the world through screens: windows, books, television, film; coats, hats, and mufflers.[13]

She goes on to describe her experience of taking up daily running.

> I felt the different textures underfoot, tarmac, gravel, grass firm and muddy, snow. I watched the park grow as spring became summer, in different light and different weather. Wind

and rain were simply that – cold and wet against the skin, bracing, not something to huddle up against. I felt the seasons change as shoots appeared, then leaves emerged emerald green, then darker in summer, then brown and gold in the autumn. . . .

Exercising the body is a positive discipline, in contrast with the negative discipline of dieting . . . once the body has become accustomed to exercise, a run, a dance session, a yoga class is something to look forward to: a freedom, not a restriction.

Much of the joy of slimming, if it exists at all, is in arriving at the goal: achieving weight loss, becoming fitter, and feeling more comfortable with one's body. The process of slimming itself yields a masochistic kind of pleasure, coming more from the knowledge of having survived a difficult obstacle course than from the act of changing one's eating habits. Survival can depend on many factors – self-confidence, self-knowledge, highly supportive family and friends, belief in one's ability to complete the course, and probably many others.

Change is never easy. We are all bound by old habits and often overestimate our capacity for major change. It is all too easy for an attempt at slimming to turn from an attempt to find joy and happiness to a recipe for misery and despair, repeated over and over again as the sufferer repeats the same mistakes. Yet changing one's behaviour in the direction of pursuing a healthier life can be immensely rewarding. Success for some people is a matter of finding the right recipe for change, and once the change has been made, there is no going back.

Chapter Six

THE DARK SIDE OF DIETING

The recipe for successful slimming eludes many people. This is not for want of trying, however, as a very great number of women believe themselves to be overweight and are often dieting.

The importance of successful dieting varies from one individual to another and depends largely on what the reasons were for dieting in the first place.

For some people the wish to be slimmer is secondary to other concerns, about family, friends, or career. For others it is of prime importance, pushing all other considerations out of the way. These people take very seriously the attitude that to be fat is to be ugly, unacceptable, and demonstrates to the world a lack of self-control, if not gluttony. Dieting may come to represent a way to succeed in the world, a way to take control of one's life. I remember an occasion when my headmistress had summoned me to her office after an inspection of my classroom at school. 'A taidy desk means a taidy mind', she declared triumphantly, as if she had just discovered the meaning of existence. Ever since then I have thought it odd the way people make glib connections between outward appearance and inner state; but time and again I have seen people who worry about their weight making similar connections: a tidy figure means a tidy life, or, more commonly, 'If only I were slim, all my problems would be solved'. So, taken to its extreme, losing weight can mean to some people a way of proving themselves to the rest of the world.

The experience of failure, therefore, can mean anything from mild disappointment for one person to crippling despair for another.

BREAKING THE DIET

Diets fail for many reasons. Often they supply inadequate nourishment and depend for their effect on starvation. Sometimes people are misguided about how much food they need and are eating too much to go into negative energy balance. More often than not, the diet comes to an end because the dieter relapses, stops keeping to the diet for perhaps only a short while, but then cannot avoid returning to old ways of eating.

Some people draw an analogy between inability to keep to a diet and addiction to substances such as alcohol, drugs, or smoking. While food in general is unlikely to be addictive, it is possible that foods containing large amounts of sugar can lead to a desire to carry on eating even if we are not hungry so that the analogy may be useful, especially for people who have what is commonly known as a 'sweet tooth'.

An American psychologist, Alan Marlatt, has categorized the situations which most commonly lead to relapse in people with addictions. He asked a group of 327 people from various abstinence programmes what were the main things that made them relapse.[1] Included in his group were twenty-nine women attending an outpatient weight-reduction programme. He defined relapse where the women were concerned as 'uncontrolled eating for a twenty-four hour period' during which the women did not use any of the practical weight-loss techniques they had been taught in the clinic. Thus they may have been very similar to any other woman who goes off her diet.

Marlatt and his colleagues were able to categorize relapse situations based on what they were told by all these people. They found that in general about half are triggered by intrapersonal events, things which come from within the person such as fear, anxiety, feeling pain, or simply having an 'urge' to do whatever it is they are trying to avoid; and half are triggered by interpersonal events, such as social pressure, or being upset by someone. Where the dieters were concerned, a third of relapses were triggered by negative emotions, such as frustration or depression, not necessarily to do with anyone else. Ten per cent were caused by social pressure, for example someone offering them food; another 10 per cent were caused by urges and temptations; 14 per cent were caused by conflict with other people; and a surprising 28 per cent were caused by feeling happy in a social situation.

Twenty-nine women in one weight-reduction programme are by no means representative of dieters at large, but other dieters might recognize the similarity between these situations and those which so often trigger them personally to loosen their control over their diet and eat something they believe is forbidden to them. As we have seen in Chapter 4, stress can trigger overeating in some people, and just feeling that one has overeaten can lead to more eating. So it is not only the relapse itself that is important but also what it means to the dieter to have slipped up.

Failed dieters live continually with the spectre of guilt. For the person who longs to be slim, who feels that her very happiness depends on it, each guilty relapse episode is just one more proof of failure. After all, everyone else can do it (can they?), the magazines and books say it is possible (is it?), so why am I so weak and incapable of doing such a small simple thing?

DIETING AND DEPRESSION

Many obese or overweight people are perfectly happy and well-adjusted. However, many others are depressed: not always despairingly, hopelessly depressed, the way people are when they need psychiatric help; but certainly they experience frequent periods of sad mood, feeling irritable, or are perhaps more tense and anxious than usual. Sometimes it is difficult to disentangle which comes first, being depressed because one is fat or being fat because one is depressed.

Some people may become fat because they are depressed. It has been suggested that fatness serves as a protection from personal difficulties. Certainly there are many people who eat more and grow fat when they are stressed or depressed, and the weight problem can come to outweigh in significance whatever reason they had for being stressed in the first place. The original problem, perhaps difficulties getting on with a spouse, apparently insoluble conflicts with parents complicated by feelings of being inadequate in some way, gets literally buried under one overriding demand – the wish to be slim.

Some writers have tried to explain depression in dieters by suggesting that being fat protects them from the world, from feeling sad; hence losing weight results in the loss of a protective coating and makes them more vulnerable to feeling depressed. However, this seems unlikely as in most cases it is only the failed dieters who feel so depressed. Many people are simply depressed because they feel fat and cannot lose weight. Conversely, people who diet successfully feel progressively happier as the pounds fall off. People drop out of diet programmes not because losing weight has made them depressed but because they cannot lose weight.

There is no doubt that dieting itself can make some people feel extremely miserable. Many dieters face devastating changes in the way they feel about food and about being fat. They begin to feel hungry all the time, even after eating; they become obsessed by thinking about food, what they have eaten today, what they will eat tomorrow. They weigh themselves once, perhaps twice or more in a day, and come to depend for their peace of mind on every slight fluctuation of the scales. They recalculate time and time again how much weight they can expect to lose by such and such a date, and when their targets are not reached, they make the calculations all over again.

Some people diet very strictly for a few days, often eating nothing for breakfast, followed by sundry 'diet' snacks, a tub of cottage cheese, a yoghurt, crispbreads, grapefruit. Overcome by hunger, and pressured by other people or by stress, they succumb to a large meal or a 'forbidden' food. The diet is broken. At best the dieter puts the lapse behind him/her and begins again. At worst, the lapse turns into a full-blown binge, and is followed by a rush to consume all the foods which for so many days or weeks have been forbidden. A leap on to the scales confirms an instant weight gain. Of course overeating does not result in weight gain pound for pound. If the extra food eaten is mainly carbohydrate – bread, cakes, sugary foods – much of the gained weight is due to the replacement of the glycogen store with its associated water (see also p. 34); but the failed dieter sees only the testimony of the scales, and all seems, and therefore is indeed, lost.

DIET AND METABOLISM

The problem is compounded because when we first go on a diet and are eating less than we were before, our metabolic rate drops. This means that we need even less fuel than before to keep us going. When we stop dieting, metabolic rate rises again, but appears to take longer to get back to its original level. Each time we cut down what we eat, metabolic rate falls more quickly. Therefore if we diet repeatedly, our metabolic rate falls each time and may not have the chance to return to its original level; so with each successive attempt at dieting, losing weight may become progressively more difficult.

The less we eat, the lower our metabolic rate falls. Also, if we lose weight at the rate of about two pounds per week, most of what we lose is fat. However, if we lose weight faster, the body begins to use up not just fat but lean tissue. At a rate of weight loss of about six pounds a week, we could be losing as much as half the weight lost in lean tissue.[2] You may be saying, 'So what? As long as I lose weight, who cares what it is made up of? It all looks the same.' The reason it does matter is that when you regain weight, it is fat that is gained first. This means that you can end up with a higher proportion of fat to lean tissue than you had before. Basal metabolic rate is dependent on how much lean tissue you have, not how much fat. Whether you lose mostly fat or mostly lean tissue may not affect the way you look, but if you end up with a higher proportion of fat to lean tissue than you had before, your metabolic rate will be lower, and you will need to eat less than you did before to stay the same weight without gaining. Hence when you try dieting again it will be that much harder.

Another problem that dieters may cause for themselves relates to the pattern of their eating. The pattern of the person described above who skips breakfast, then eats little else throughout the day, is not uncommon. Another pattern is to eat little or nothing at all during the day and then have a meal in the evening. Many diets, and some professional dietitians, stipulate that you must 'have breakfast' on a diet. This sounds over-finicky and many people resent being told when they should eat. There is, however, some sense in it, as researchers have found that eating more often can have the effect of ensuring the least possible drop in metabolic rate. For example, a group of researchers compared the basal metabolic rates of 208 obese patients with their meal-eating patterns.[3] There were five meal patterns: nothing eaten until supper; lunch and supper only; three meals a day; three meals plus up to three snacks; and three meals plus three or more snacks. There was a strong relationship between basal metabolic rate and number of meals or snacks eaten and the researchers concluded that people who skip breakfast have significantly lower basal metabolic rates than people who eat three or more meals a day. So whether you feel you can stomach breakfast or not, it may be preferable to spread eating over the whole day rather than eating only once or twice. (Provided of course that you do not eat more altogether than you did before going on the diet!) There is also another advantage in this: if you eat at frequent intervals you are less likely to suffer extreme deprivation and find yourself unable to stop whenever you do finally allow yourself to eat.

STARVATION AND ITS SYMPTOMS

Deprivation, both real and imagined, is one of the major problems of a long-term diet. The problem is not just psychological, as some researchers in Minnesota found when they conducted an experiment to investigate the effects of long-term starvation during the Second World War.[4] They asked thirty-six male conscientious objectors to take part in an experiment to see what happens to people when they undergo starvation. The men ate normally during the first three months of the experiment while their behaviour, eating patterns, and personality were studied. They were then put on strict diets where their normal intakes were cut by half for a period of three months. Afterwards they went through a three-month period of 'rehabilitation' when they were reintroduced to eating normal amounts of food. These men were thoughtful people who had objected on moral grounds to joining the war as fighters, but who were keen to help in any other way they could. Therefore they were conscientious about sticking to their diets. They were also people who had previously had no particular interest in food or dieting.

What happened in the experiment suggests that the effects of severely reducing one's intake are far reaching. Food became the main topic of conversation, reading, and daydreams for almost all of the men. Men who had previously had no particular interest in food and cooking became fascinated by cookery and menus, and about two-thirds of them started to read cookbooks and collect recipes. About half-way through the semi-starvation period thirteen of the men expressed an interest in taking up cooking after the experiment was over. A few of them even planned to become chefs! Many of the men found it impossible to keep to the diet. They ate secretly on impulse and felt guilty afterwards. Psychologically they became more worrying and prone to feeling depressed, they had difficulty in concentrating, and they began to withdraw from other people and become less sociable.

At the end of the semi-starvation period, the men's personalities reverted to normal. However, very many of them continued to have problems with eating. They were now allowed to eat whatever they liked, but they continued to want more than they were given and to be preoccupied with food and how they would eat it. Some of them reported that their hunger pangs were even worse than before. Some had cravings for certain foods: mainly sweets (ice-cream and pastries), dairy products (milk, eggs, cheese), and nuts. Three weeks after the special diet had ended, at least four of the men found themselves unable to feel full up after eating and wanted to eat more even though their stomachs were full to bursting; and many of them snacked between meals. Another four weeks later, ten of the fifteen men who were still in touch with the researchers had become so concerned about their weight that they had put themselves on a reducing diet. A few were continuing to eat 'prodigious' quantities of food and had gained weight. Three months after the end of the starvation phase, food was still a major concern of fifteen out of twenty-four men.

These effects of starvation are fairly powerful. Of course because this was an experiment the circumstances surrounding it were very abnormal. However, the calorie allowance was not dissimilar from that of many very stringent diets; and the experiment is of particular interest because it described the experience of men, who are not usually greatly concerned about dieting and weight. These men experienced thoughts and feelings remarkably similar to those of people who feel deprived on a slimming diet. What is more, the experience of dieting itself engendered in these men a concern about weight and diet which they had not felt previously. In other words, very strict dieting can itself cause the dieter to develop a concern about weight and diet which they have not experienced before. Moreover, the concern continued to be a problem for up to eight months after the 'diet' was over.

Worrying about weight can lead to strict dieting which can for some people lead to further preoccupation. Starvation can result in a tendency to binge and therefore undo all the good work, and therefore back into a cycle of dieting, continuous overeating, and dieting again.

BINGE EATING

Binge eating has become a subject of major interest in the last few years. For one thing, there are now probably very few people who would not admit to binge eating sometimes. This is fine if it means that we can all feel less guilty and more relaxed about what we choose to eat; but there is another side to the coin. The word 'binge' is now so commonly used that its definition has become very broad. Essentially, a binge is eating a large amount of food in a short space of time even after the point at which one is no longer aware of feeling hungry, and eating in an uncontrolled way so that stopping is difficult. For one person a binge might constitute having three meals one after the other followed by a packet of biscuits; but for many other people a binge may be indicated by having two slices of bread too many (too many by whose standards?). As we have seen, binge eating can be triggered off by long periods of deprivation. It is almost as though our bodies are telling us that we have not been eating enough and need to catch up, even if we are not hungry now. However, binges can also be triggered by the mere thought that one has eaten too much. There is a danger therefore in dieters being too hard on themselves: in working to keep their intake under some ideal limit, they cannot resist exceeding it; when this happens, they may find themselves having a real binge. Hence they feel guilty, they make a new attempt to keep to a strict diet, only to find themselves more deeply trapped in a cycle of overeating, binge eating, guilt, dieting, and overeating again.

How many people binge eat?

In recent years there has been a great deal of interest in the phenomenon of binge eating. About 50 per cent of overweight people have admitted in some surveys to binge eating at least once a week; and binge eating is a problem which can prevent people from benefiting from weight-loss programmes unless there is help built in to overcome it.

Far more interest, however, has surrounded the phenomenon of the person of normal weight who binges. Several surveys have been carried out which suggest that it is a problem which occurs particularly in young women. Many of the surveys have been conducted with college students. In one survey in New England, for example, 631 women and 276 men returned questionnaires out of a total of 800 and 400 respectively sent out.[5] Only 10 per cent of the respondents were overweight, but 50 per cent of the women and 13 per cent of the men thought they were overweight. Nearly a quarter of the women admitted that they were binge eating on amounts of at least 1,000 calories at a time, at least once a week on average. College students are not the only people with the problem however. In a survey of 369 women attending a family planning clinic in England, one-quarter of the women admitted to binge eating at least once a week; and one-fifth of the women thought that they had an eating problem. In fact most of the women were at or around normal weight for their height, but 60 per cent felt persistently overweight and on average the women wanted to lose eleven pounds.[6]

The extent to which people have problems with binge eating appears to relate very closely to how far they feel themselves to be overweight, how often they are dieting, and how far weight is a worry to them. Often too, it appears to relate to images people have of themselves, how self-confident they are. This may be because, for the majority of normal-weight dieters, dieting is a way of demonstrating that one is in control in a world that puts a premium on conveying a certain image. Only the very self-assured woman can say 'I'm happy with the way I am' and resist the temptation to be carried along on the dieting tide. Many other less confident women may be drawn into dieting needlessly. Compulsive eating may well begin as part of the body's response to being deprived of adequate nourishment but may rapidly become a source of shame and a cause of downward spiralling self-esteem.

'DIETING DISEASES'

While binge eating is fairly common and as such may be considered quite normal, a fraction of people have problems with it that have serious effects on their lives. Some people suffer for many years with a serious eating problem without ever seeking help. Even those who do ask for help have often had the problem for several years before they are able to do anything about it. One of the difficulties may be that until recently people with problems around food have had to suffer in silence because they simply were not aware that other people suffer too.

Bulimia nervosa

For between one and three in a hundred young women, problems

75

with binge eating and its consequences have come to dominate their daily lives and fill their thoughts. Even their social and work lives can become affected by the need to binge and its consequences, and their feelings about how their lives and personal relationships are going are coloured by whether they have had a 'good' day or a 'bad' day.

This is the phenomenon called 'bulimia' or, more commonly in Britain, 'bulimia nervosa'. People who suffer with this problem are terrified of gaining weight or becoming fat, and they have frequent uncontrollable urges to eat. Feeling ashamed of their abnormal pattern of eating, they often eat alone, in private, and may succeed in hiding the problem for many years even from loved ones and people living with them. This can require enormous effort on the part of sufferers, as in order to conceal their eating habits from others they may have to confine their eating to places away from home, for example walking along the street on the way home from work, or eating in the car; or they may have to find ways of secretly replacing large amounts of food eaten at home.

In between bouts of overeating they diet strictly, or attempt to counteract the effects of overeating by making themselves vomit or by taking laxatives. Unfortunately, none of these methods is an effective means of weight control. Severe restriction, as we have seen, is difficult to keep up, and can lead only to problems with being able to eat a normal amount of food without gaining weight or at worst to further binge eating.

Purging – the use of vomiting or laxatives – is not an effective solution to a weight-control problem. The idea of vomiting after having eaten too much is not new. The Romans used to do it, and even had special 'vomitoria'. Some people have the idea themselves after eating a particularly large amount of food and perhaps feeling very sick. Vomiting serves to relieve them and hence may become a habit. Other people may have begun the habit initially at the suggestion of a friend or relative. Others have read about it in a book or magazine. It is for this reason that I mention the problem here, as it may be useful to detail its disadvantages for any sufferer who feels tempted to consider it as a solution to their own eating problem.

Regular vomiting can cause serious medical problems. Apart from looking red-eyed and suffering minor problems such as the bursting of tiny blood vessels around the eyes, sufferers often develop problems with their teeth. They may also develop swollen salivary glands, which can only exacerbate the feeling of being fat as they cause the face to look 'puffy'. Worse than that, essential minerals are lost in vomit, and sufferers can experience symptoms such as muscle weakness, headache, tiredness, and palpitations. Some people have suffered kidney problems and cardiac irregularities.

Neither is taking laxatives the answer to an eating problem. By the time the food has gone through the stomach and intestines and into the colon, most of what was to be absorbed by the body has already been absorbed. The sufferer feels thinner but only because the diarrhoea caused by the laxatives has made her dehydrated: in other words, most of the loss is water and as soon as she eats or drinks again, the loss is automatically made up over the next few days.

Psychologically too, purging is a very unsatisfactory solution to an eating problem. Like binging, it can become a habit. In the absence of any other way of controlling their eating, some binge eaters find themselves in a vicious circle where they are having to purge in order to deal with their overeating.

Nancy, for example, came to see me with a binge-eating problem. She was starving herself all day, and in the evenings eating whatever she could find in the refrigerator – bread, ice-cream, left-over cakes. Day after day she would vomit to rid herself of this food, and promise herself that tomorrow she would eat only salads and 'healthy' foods. Once she had discovered a way of ridding herself of the excess calories, however, she was able to delude herself that she could make a fresh start, and so altering her eating habits became even more difficult.

Getting into the habit of purging can also lead to problems with maintaining a steady weight on a normal amount of food. Alison came to see me after she had lost a great deal of weight very fast, through keeping herself on a strict diet. She was terrified of regaining her lost weight and for some months had been taking several laxatives at least twice a week, whenever she had to eat socially with friends and therefore could not stick to her self-prescribed ration of crackers and cottage cheese. Naturally, whenever she did eat a normal meal, her stomach would feel big and she would appear to gain weight. The laxatives she took made her feel very ill, but she was prepared to take them as they also made her feel slimmer. In fact they were making her dehydrated, and gradually she continued to gain weight. Frightened by her apparent weight gain, she ate very little all day and a small meal in the evenings for weeks at a time. No doubt her metabolic rate was dropping as her intake went down and she was having to exist on a decreasing amount of food. It was only through coming to accept that she might have to regain a small amount of her former weight while learning to eat normally again that she was able to give up the laxatives and allow herself to eat a little more throughout the day.

Descriptions of people with bulimia usually emphasize their normal weight; however, both fat people and very thin people can suffer in the same way, often as a corollary to strict dieting which they are no longer able to keep up.

Anorexia nervosa

This is the disorder often known as the 'slimming disease'. Sufferers usually begin with conscious dieting to lose weight, although only about one-third of them were previously overweight. They begin dieting perhaps because they have been teased, or perhaps along with a specific life change such as starting work or college, or starting a first serious relationship with a boyfriend.[7] The dieting turns into a 'relentless pursuit of slimness' fired by a terror of becoming fat;[8] and the sufferer loses so much weight as to become emaciated.[9] Sufferers are usually in their adolescence, but may develop the disorder at any time between the ages of 12 and 35 years,[10] and a few have been known to develop it even later. Most are female, but about one in sixteen are male.

Anorexia nervosa sufferers keep their weight down by severely restricting what they eat and often by taking excessive amounts of exercise, running, jogging, 'working out'. Some find themselves giving in to urges to binge, and try to counteract the effects of the binges by vomiting and purging.

Some of the symptoms of anorexia nervosa are strikingly similar to those experienced by people undergoing starvation, described on p. 72. While declaring to the world that they are not hungry, many sufferers feel hungry all the time and think about food constantly. They may become fascinated by cooking and preparing beautiful meals for other people, although they cannot allow themselves to eat; they may become obsessed by calories and some develop a great interest in health foods. When they do eat, they may pick at their

THE DARK SIDE OF DIETING

food, pushing it around on the plate for ages before finishing it.

Dieting and eating disorder

Some groups of people appear to be more prone to developing eating disorders than others. The need to diet in itself or to avoid eating particular foods appears to put certain people at risk.

One group of people who have to be very careful of their diet are insulin-dependent diabetics. They have to control their diet so that their need for insulin remains steady. They cannot cope with rapid rises in blood sugar, and so are usually advised to limit the amount of snack and sugary foods they eat. Therefore they have to eat regular, well-balanced meals, they may have to count calories or carbohydrate units in order to keep their weight down, and often they have a list of 'forbidden' foods. Despite, or perhaps because of, the chronic and life-threatening nature of the disease, not everyone is able to do exactly as they are told by the doctors. Some people find it very difficult to stick to their strict regime, and find themselves binging and purging, and sometimes manipulating their diabetes to control their weight. In fact, eating disorders may be twice as common in diabetic adolescents as in non-diabetic adolescents.[11]

Another group of people who suffer a high incidence of eating disorders is the group of people who need to be slim for cosmetic reasons, and for reasons connected with their work. Recently, for example, people are becoming concerned about the increasing tendency of athletes, both male and female, to develop eating disorders. Runners in particular sometimes appear similar to anorexics in their behaviour, possibly as a result of the constant need to starve themselves; and other athletes who need to stay within a certain weight class so that they can ensure their place in a particular team can have similar problems.

The prevalence of anorexic attitudes and even of the disorder itself is higher in groups of dancers, modelling students, and beauty therapy students than in the general population.[12,13] These are people on whom there is a great pressure to be slim, as otherwise they may do less well in the competition for jobs where a sylph-like figure is at a premium.

Is dieting the sole cause of eating disorders?

In describing the symptoms of bulimia and anorexia nervosa I do not wish to imply that they are the inevitable consequences of strict dieting. As we have seen, some 50 per cent of women are dieting at any one time and very many women have problems connected with food, dieting, and weight. Serious eating disorders, while on the increase, are still fairly rare: less than one in a hundred women suffer from anorexia nervosa, perhaps two in a hundred have bulimia nervosa, and up to one in five have problems which, though serious, are not life-threatening.

Starvation, while clearly a trigger for major eating problems, is unlikely to be the sole cause of these problems. The symptoms of anorexia nervosa in athletes can be reversed with help which involves education about the problem and instructions about gradual weight loss. Similarly, ballet students who develop the symptoms of anorexia nervosa do not necessarily continue to suffer with the disease to the detriment of their careers.[14]

One of the chief factors that appears to distinguish consistently between people who develop serious long-term eating problems and people who do not is that of self-esteem. Compared with other women and adolescents, people with bulimia and anorexia nervosa consistently describe themselves as being low in self-confidence and insecure about their relationships with other people. In addition, they are often unhappy with their body image, in that they see themselves as fat, or believe that a part of them is too fat and needs to be changed so as to make them look acceptable in the eyes of other people.

These problems in themselves, however, while understandable as a context for dieting, cannot fully explain the development of a serious life-threatening disorder. What is more likely is that several factors combine to create a setting for a serious eating problem.

One of these factors may be that of family background. Many clinical descriptions of anorexia nervosa and bulimia imply that sufferers frequently come from families where relationships are disturbed or are overclose so that the child has been unable to distinguish her own needs and wants from those of her family and has therefore not developed her own clear identify separate from theirs. As adulthood approaches, she is expected to make all kinds of decisions for which she is ill prepared: about career, about relationships. An additional factor which may be important is the nature of women's position in today's society. It has been suggested by the feminist movement that in this day and age the life decisions faced by women are particularly difficult. Young women are in the impossible position of having to be all things to many people: intelligent and educated, sexually liberated, and able to compete with male aggression if they wish to succeed in the career stakes. Yet at the same time in order to be acceptable in society they must appear passively attractive, good at 'home-making', warm, all attributes which are at odds with the idea that women and men have an equal right to demand from each other and share as equal partners in life. One feminist writer expresses the dilemma as follows:

> There is continuous pressure on us, for even when our behaviour does get the okay, we are never really sure if we have succeeded or if the rules have changed. For example, we cut our hair in the latest bob only to read that long hair is back, or we stay at home to bring up the children only to be told that it wasn't necessary and why hadn't we got a job and contributed to the housekeeping? We are kept constantly on our toes, dancing to somebody else's tune which isn't even clear to us.[15]

In this context dieting can become the stage for acting out conflicts that are central to a woman's life. Everywhere the successful dieter is admired. Even the anorexic is secretly admired for her rigid self-control. One mother of an 18-year-old anorexic, while complaining that she could not persuade her 'child' to eat, mentioned that her daughter, so self-conscious about what she perceived as her fat thighs, would sit on the beach wearing her track suit pants. 'But she's a very striking looking girl; most people would give anything to have legs like that,' said her mother.

We cannot control other people, or our relationships with them. An adolescent may face the additional problems of low self-confidence and feelings of ambivalence about exactly how to be in the world. Food, because it is such an essential commodity in our lives, can continue from babyhood to hold a central place in the way we demonstrate our relationship with the world. Therefore the choice between eating and not eating can become a natural focus for life's problems.

How then can we diet without risking problems with eating or developing a lifelong obsession with food and weight? The answer to this question is complicated. In the first place it is vital to address the question of the reasons for dieting. Are we protecting our health or are we using a diet as a way to protect ourselves from real or imagined criticism? If dieting is used as a form of self-improvement, we have to be very sure that a slim figure is really the improvement that is needed. So many times, the underlying message put across by a dieter is that she is unhappy with herself and wishes to change. It is all too tempting to believe that all will be well if only you are slim.

Second, once having made the decision to diet, dieters need to be aware that success is not achieved simply by the desire to be slim or by an extended period of semi-starvation; and moreover that tackling a diet in this way can have negative physiological and psychological effects which at best are temporarily painful and at worst can throw them into dietary chaos.

Chapter Seven

EATING TO LIVE

Dieting does not suit everyone. Perhaps the worst aspect of dieting and the way it is currently portrayed is the flavour of self-deprivation that goes with it: the notions of guilt and punishment, with dieting as a kind of mortification of the flesh and eating as a guilty reward, to be paid for later by dieting again.

Eating is of course rewarding to all of us, as without food we die; but when food is our main source of satisfaction and weight a central preoccupation, then all is not well. As we have seen in Chapter 5, the people who fare best when dieting are those who are able to make permanent alterations in their eating habits: they are usually also people who can find satisfaction from things in their lives other than food; and whose life-styles can accommodate a change in their relationship with food.

In a sense, successful dieters are often people who are able to shift the emphasis on food in their homes away from the idea that certain foods are to be eaten only rarely as 'treats' and towards the idea of more healthy eating for the family as a whole.

EATING FOR HEALTH

My intention in this book is not primarily to advocate this or that method of dieting, or to recommend specific items of food. However, it may be relevant to say something about recent dietary advice and to convey the message that healthy eating can be a habit worth getting into. For months at a time many of us are used to consuming items which have little nutritional value: pre-packaged processed foods containing more sugar, salt, and fats than we need, high-calorie snack foods. It is only when we put on weight and decide to diet that we take ourselves in hand and start to opt for fresh fruit and vegetables, lean meat, and fish. Hence the common complaint of dieters that keeping to a diet is expensive, and the tendency of many dieters to cook one thing for themselves, and an alternative meal for their families. Certain foods become relabelled as foods to be eaten when 'on a diet', so adding to the dieter's experience of isolation, of being excluded, even deprived. There can be few experiences more galling for some overweight people than sitting at a meal with other family members, all eating large portions of fried potato chips, while gnawing their way through a plateful of salad.

As an alternative to the notion of being either 'on' or 'off' a reducing diet, it may make more sense to adopt a way of eating that makes us more likely to stay in good health and less likely to need to 'diet' in the first place. Then, if it does become necessary to lose weight, this can be a more or less painless exercise, involving us simply in cutting down what we normally eat rather than having to adopt a style of eating which is altogether alien to us and therefore difficult to maintain.

WHY SHOULD IT MATTER WHAT WE EAT?

You may be asking why on earth it should matter what you eat if you do not have a medical problem which means that you have to exclude certain items or if you are within a reasonable weight range for your height. A very common complaint of the person who needs to diet to lose weight is that other people can eat what they like. The most bitter complaints are not about things like extra large bowls of soup, helpings of meat, or pounds of fruit and vegetables. They are invariably about the kind of food that is most to be avoided on a slimming diet. Here are some examples of the kind of comment I am referring to.

A young woman who works in an office:

It's so unfair. They can eat what they like. All day long the other girls eat crisps, bars of chocolate, and have chips with their lunch while I just have to keep saying 'no'. Then sometimes when it's a birthday they bring in cream cakes and all day long the blessed things are sitting there in front of me. Then it's very hard to resist. After all, I'd feel pretty silly saying, 'Please would you take those away, they're upsetting me!'

A mother of two teenage sons who does all the providing and cooking for the family:

> They always seem to be hungry. I don't know where they put it. A big cooked breakfast: bacon, sausages, eggs, the lot. Then sandwiches, chocolate bars and crisps for lunch, a big cooked meal in the evening. I always have to cook something different for myself. They love chips and complain if there aren't any. Then I usually do a pudding as well.

A mother of two small children:

> They love cakes and chocolates. As long as they've eaten their supper, I can't see any reason why they should not have any. After all, they're not fat, they take after their father, lucky things, skinny as a rake.

A man who works for an advertising company:

> After work everyone goes to the pub for a drink. I know I shouldn't drink on my diet, but I only have a couple of pints. It's very difficult to say 'no' when everyone else is drinking, makes you feel unsociable. Then I get hungry, so sometimes if I know I'm going to get home late I have a packet of crisps. That's OK because it's got less calories than peanuts.

These comments always imply a certain degree of envy. They also carry certain assumptions about what it is to eat normally. One of these is that it is preferable to be sociable and eat the same things as everyone else. A second assumption is that if the person was not 'on a diet' they too would be free to eat in the same way. A third assumption is that if the dieter is the person preparing the food, they should continue to provide exactly the kinds of meal for their families that they were providing before.

However, we all surely have the right to eat what we like and when we like regardless of the opinions of friends or colleagues and to accept or refuse food when it is offered. Second, as we have seen, people eat what they are used to, and they can get used to a variety of different kinds of diet, as anyone who has done some foreign travel will know. This means that the person who buys, cooks, and serves the food for the family has a great deal of control over what goes on to the table and into the mouths of the family members. There is no need for anyone of whatever age, and however slim, to eat as part of their diet a high percentage of refined foods, fats, or sugars, or to consume large amounts of alcohol. In fact recent medical opinion has suggested that the kind of food that we eat can have important effects on our long-term health.

In 1983 the NACNE Report was published. This was a report written by a committee commissioned by the government to summarize all the available information about nutrition and health.[1]

The report questioned the validity of the 'balanced diet' as we know it. Until recently, we have been told that the best diet is a balanced diet, which means that we should be eating some proteins, fats, carbohydrates, minerals and vitamins in our diet. Foods were categorized arbitrarily, so that cheese, for example, which also contains a great deal of fat, was regarded as a protein food. Sugar, which gives energy but little else, was considered acceptable as long as it was 'balanced' in the diet by other nutrients. Now the emphasis is less on what we need to eat, because many single food items can contain several nutrients, than on what we need to avoid eating because of the harmful effects on our health of eating certain foods.

There is increasing evidence that some diseases are diet related. They may be caused by eating too much of a particular food or by not eating enough of some foods. Some of the evidence comes from looking at the relationship between consumption and disease in different countries of the world and in groups of people with similar life-styles but different eating habits. In the west, and particularly in Britain, we have a higher level of consumption of saturated fats, salt, and sugar than in the rest of the world and also the highest incidence of premature death from heart disease, and certain cancers. On the other hand, doctors have found that people with high intakes of dietary fibre (found in fruit, vegetables, pulses, and grains) are less likely to develop these diseases than people with low-fibre intakes. Thus, diets high in fibre may protect us from disease. In the east, fibre in the form of grains and pulses is often the mainstay of diet, and diseases like heart disease, certain cancers, and diseases of the intestines, are comparatively rare. Table 1 illustrates the relationship between over- and under-consumption of foods and disease.

In addition to the associations indicated in the table, several other links are currently being identified between diet and certain diseases. For example, it has been suggested that there may be links between fat intake and rheumatoid arthritis, and multiple sclerosis. Another

86

Table 1 Suggested links between foods and disease. Adapted from: *The Great British Diet*, The British Dietetic Association and Dr Andrew Stanway, 1985, Century Publishing

Disease	Associated with too much	Associated with too little
Tooth decay	Sugar	Fibre
Digestive system:		
constipation		Fibre
diverticular disease		Fibre
irritable bowel		Fibre
hiatus hernia		Fibre
appendicitis		Fibre
cancer of the colon	Fat	Fibre
gall bladder disease	Calorie intake, fat	Fibre
Heart and blood vessels:		
heart disease	Fat, calorie intake	Fibre
high blood pressure	Calorie intake, salt, fat	Fibre (?)
stroke	Calorie intake, salt, fat	
Breast cancer	Fat, alcohol?	
Stomach cancer	Salt	
Diabetes, maturity onset	Calorie intake	
Liver disease	Alcohol	

area, somewhat controversial still in the extent to which it can be taken seriously, is the topic of food allergy and the relationship between foods or food additives and behaviour or mood.[2]

Taking into account the now apparent dangers of our western eating style, the NACNE Report made several recommendations for change. Incidentally, the authors of the report were not alone in their opinion that we need to modify our diet. Some years previously, a report had been published in the USA which made similar suggestions.[3]

The recommendations of the NACNE Report were very broadly as follows. We should cut our intake of fats, in particular of saturated fats.[4] We should cut our consumption of sugar by half (this also means cutting the number of sugary snacks we take). We should increase the amount of fibre in our diet – wholegrains, cereals, vegetables, and fruit. We should cut down the amount of salt we take. We should drink less alcohol. We should take less animal protein and more plant protein. We should decrease our intake of processed foods and eat more whole, fresh foods.[5]

At this point, many readers would question what all this has got to do with dieting. Items such as bread, potatoes, beans, and pasta are all items which traditionally people on diets have avoided. However, it has been suggested by some people that on the contrary such foods might help with long-term weight loss and maintenance. One reason for this is that high-carbohydrate, high-fibre diets take longer to eat and therefore we may feel more full up and satisfied afterwards; another reason is that some high-fibre foods delay the rate at which the stomach empties so that we may feel full for longer.[6]

Making changes in one's diet to follow recent dietary advice is not always easy. Moreover the exact nature of the ideal diet has been a subject of some controversy. Some members of the British Dietetic Association undertook a survey of 472 adults including 289 dietitians to see how viable the changes advocated by NACNE might be.[7] They then described the results of their survey in a book called *The Great British Diet*, although they were careful to emphasize that the ideas they were putting across were their own and not necessarily representative of the policy of the British Dietetic Association. The participants had to keep detailed records of their food intake for one week, during which they ate their normal diet, and again in a second week during which they were instructed to eat following the guidelines suggested by NACNE; 351 people managed to complete the second week of record-keeping. Of these, 47 per cent said that the new eating pattern could become a way of life, 27 per cent were uncertain, and 26 per cent said that they did not think they could keep it up.

The interesting thing about the study is that the participants included a large percentage of dietitians, people who are trained in good nutrition. If the changes created difficulties for these people then how much more difficult might they be for those of us without any nutritional knowledge? In fact those things which the participants found most difficult were possibly the very things that would cause problems for the rest of us. For example, they missed sweets, snacks, chips, fats, and dairy products. We cook and eat the things we have been used to eating for a long time, and changing our buying, cooking, and eating habits is not something we can expect to be able to do overnight. Also, the food took extra time to prepare. One possible reason for this of course is that more time had to be spent poring over recipe books! Another problem for some people was the lack of suitable foods in restaurants and at work, the lack of suitable convenience foods, and the lack of between-meal snacks.

Much available convenience or snack food contains a great deal of added sugar or salt, or is high in saturated fats.

Nevertheless, it is possible to make changes if they are introduced to the family in a gradual way, perhaps even one at a time. Some of the suggestions made by the authors of *The Great British Diet* are worth repeating here. They suggest that changes are gradual, in particular in relation to eating more food that is high in fibre, to avoid the possibility of sudden increases in stools, especially in small children. They suggest that mainly nutritious foods are kept at home, so that food cravings have to be satisfied with bread, cereals, and fruit rather than cakes, biscuits, and confectionery. In relation to children they make the comment that example is the best teacher. If children do not see their parents eating their way through bars of chocolate or tins of biscuits while watching TV then they will be less likely to want to do so.

FEEDING A FAMILY

Food is an emotive topic for many people. So is the subject of children. Put the two together, and you have a veritable minefield. The giving of food by a mother to her baby and the acceptance by baby of the food is a matter of crucial importance in the first few months of their relationship. Feeding her baby is one of the only material ways in which a mother can feel that she is satisfying her child and giving it love. If for some reason there is a problem which makes feeding difficult, feeding times can become fraught with emotion. A mother has to learn to recognize when her baby is hungry and when not. If baby cries, she has to distinguish between a host of possible reasons of which hunger is only one: including anger, boredom, fear, pain, or discomfort. Some parents find this very easy; others have more difficulty, and are understandably tempted to use food as a universal pacifier. In this context, many babies are often fed at inappropriate times, or with foods that they do not really need at that moment. Hence they may be perfectly adequately fed, but are not getting the chance to learn to distinguish for themselves when they are hungry and when not.

Children's eating habits change over time. Sometimes they have days when they do not feel like eating at all, at other times they want very little, and sometimes they want to eat more. This is all quite normal, but can be worrying for some parents, who find themselves getting locked into a battle of persuasion. The scenario of mother taking every item out of the refrigerator one by one and offering it to a disinterested infant is a familiar one which can all too often develop into a game in which the infant is invariably the winner. Unfortunately, it is all too easy to offer foods low in nutritional value either as a reward for eating a meal, or because parents would rather see a child eat something than nothing at all. But offering 'junk' food in this way is a mistake for several reasons.

First, while there is some evidence that we all have a tendency to like sweet things, our liking for particular foods depends on our experience. If we have never had ice-cream, we won't miss it. On the whole, children prefer the foods they are used to eating.[8]

Second, it is never a good idea to make an issue of food. As we have seen, distinguishing the feeling we call 'hunger' from other sensations is not without problems for any of us; but if left to his or her own devices, every child can learn to recognize, at least as well as humanly possible, when it is time to eat. Some parents might dispute this, as there are a few toddlers who refuse food and hence cause a great deal of upset. Indeed between 10 and 30 per cent of children under the age of 5 are described by their parents as faddy or finicky and it is common for parents to worry about how much their children are eating.[9] Very rarely, a young child may refuse to eat for a medical reason. Usually, however, a more simple explanation is likely. Either the child is simply not in need of food at that time or the reason has something to do with the way the child feels about things. This is not the same as naughtiness. Just like an adult, a child may feel less inclined to eat when upset or when not getting on well with other members of the family. Besides, eating or not eating is for a young child one of the few ways he or she has of complying or not with adult demands and therefore expressing feelings. This being the case, the best strategy is to relax, stop worrying, and let the child eat in his or her own time. As always when we are dealing with emotive problems, the most sensible solution is the most difficult to put into practice!

There is another reason why offering rewards to persuade children to eat is not a good idea in the long run. As we saw in Chapter 4, most children's liking for a particular food goes down if they are offered a reward in exchange for eating it; at the same time their liking for the reward itself goes up. Thus, for example, if parents use food rewards such as chocolates to persuade their child to eat his vegetables they could be producing exactly the opposite effect to the one they want: the child will like the vegetables even less and the chocolates more! Indeed, parents who use sweets as rewards are often the same parents who worry about how many sweets their children have.[10]

On the whole, children (and adults) like best what they are used to. Besides, they are more likely to accept novel foods if they see adults eating them.[11] Therefore the choice of what kind of food your family eats is largely up to you. This means that while it may not be possible entirely to avoid children becoming fat, or suffering ill health in later life, you have the opportunity to ensure that their diet is as healthy as possible. There will of course be times when a child will have a 'craze' for a particular food, and refuse to eat everything else. Similarly, children learn from copying each other, and can quite often develop a taste for a particular food because they have seen their friends eat it. This is all to be expected, but 'fads' do not necessarily last. So trying to influence what your children eat when they go out may cause more trouble than it is worth. They spend far more time with you and so are going to learn by your example to enjoy the foods you eat at home.

Just as important as it is to take the emotion out of food and eating situations where children are concerned, it is important for would-be dieters to do so for themselves and for other adult members of the family. How often do you reward yourself with food, treating yourself for example in compensation for a disappointment? This is not to say that there is anything intrinsically wrong with having good food, only to question the context in which it is eaten. In order to feel relaxed about food and dieting it is necessary to feel that one has the freedom to eat whatsoever one likes without fear or guilt. This also means that one has to have a certain level of satisfaction with the way one looks and the confidence to believe either that dieting is not necessary or that if attempted it will be successful. The following chapters are designed to help readers to decide whether dieting is the main issue in the first place, to develop some strategies for getting it right in the second, and finally to overcome the more serious problems which can arise when eating and emotion become inextricably linked.

Chapter Eight

COPING WITH A DIET 1: DEFINING THE PROBLEM

Many people agonize constantly about their weight. Dieting is a common activity, pursued by a great number of people who have no need to do so. Dieting of itself, however, brings few immediate rewards, even to those people for whom weight loss is crucial to their physical well-being.

Most people, when faced with a decision about taking a new path in life, give some thought to factors such as their likelihood of achieving success, the disadvantages to them of attempting the change, and what they will lose should the attempt fail. A young person who wishes to work in a bank, for example, will try to find out how much natural talent for figures he or she has; how much training is needed and how difficult it will be, and how much it will cost financially and emotionally to finish the training. In contrast, dieters often make the assumption that anyone can diet successfully and, in the absence of information about exactly what dieting will involve or a clear plan of action, begin a diet only to fail. It is possible that, unlike the person who considers working in the bank, the would-be dieter has no real choice. The choice is either to get slim or to consider oneself a failure.

There is no reason, however, why dieting should not be tackled in the same way as any other long-term plan. This means that in the first place the dieter must find out whether dieting is necessary, and whether indeed there is a choice between dieting and not dieting. Second, he or she must find out what skills or assets he or she has that will help in keeping to the diet, and what skills are lacking and need to be learned.

DO YOU REALLY NEED TO DIET?

A part of the process of deciding whether or not to diet must consist of making a judgement about how necessary it is. The word 'necessity' is usually as subjective in relation to the concept of dieting as it is in relation to how big a house we each of us need to live in comfort. While I might be happy to park my car in the street and grow flowers in pots, you might require a garage and a hundred feet of garden.

'Surely,' you may say, 'I know when I need to diet by the way my clothes fit me, or by looking at myself in the mirror.' To some extent this is true, but there is a problem here. Every day, we are confronted with images of super-slim people, wearing super-small clothes. Given that the ideal figure for women, if not always for men, is thin, we may be biased always to see ourselves as less than perfect, and in need of modification.

How overweight are you?

One way of avoiding the problems attendant on unnecessary dieting is to start with the weight tables. The Health Education Authority in Britain have taken the table devised by Professor John Garrow (see Chapter 2) and turned it around so as to make it easily readable. The table demonstrates the ranges of weight for each height and also gives some indication of the severity of different degrees of above normal weight (see Figure 3). To assess your own weight, first find out your height without shoes, and weigh yourself without clothes. Take a straight line up from your weight along the bottom of the graph and another line across from your height. Where the two lines meet tells you which range of W/H^2 your weight comes into.

If you fall into the band marked 'O', you are within the normal range of weight for your height. Slimming would be a cosmetic exercise, and would have no value as far as your health is concerned.

If your weight falls into any of the bands marked I, II, or III, you may wish to think about dieting. There are several factors, however, that you may want to take into account when deciding whether you should diet or not, especially if you fall into the mildly overweight category.

Weighing up the risks

First, you should be aware of the dangers of being overweight (see Chapter 2). At the same time, you might want to take into consideration the importance of the individual risk factors in relation to your own case: that is, for example, whether you or your family have a history of high blood pressure or diabetes. You may also want to consider whether you have other habits which may be harming your health, such as smoking or drinking alcohol on a daily basis. This is not to say that if you reduce one risk factor you can ignore the others. However, depending on how overweight you are, there may be strategies other than dieting, in particular giving up cigarettes, or perhaps reducing the stress in your life and increasing the amount of exercise you take, that will improve your health. No one can be expected to make several changes at once. If you are trying to change other habits as well as the way you eat, it is best to take things slowly and tackle the problems one by one as you are more likely to succeed the easier your task is.

Weighing up the advantages of weight loss

Another factor you should take into account is the question of why you want to lose weight. In other words, what do you expect to get out of being slimmer? Slimness is lauded as the ideal state to be. What would be the benefits to you in health terms? How much difference would it make to you socially and personally to be slimmer? How different would the attitude of other people be towards you? How far does your wish to be slimmer come from you alone, and how far does it come from other people? There is a great deal of pressure on us, and on women in particular, to be slim. This pressure is said to come largely via the media and attitudes towards fatter people in general (see pp. 25–8); but inevitably it comes through individuals too. I have often met women of normal weight who tell me that their boyfriend or fiancé would like them to be slimmer or even that an agreement to marry is dependent on the woman achieving a lower weight. Sometimes the specific weight level has been set by the girl herself, but the boyfriend goes along with the idea of not setting a wedding date until the weight has been achieved. In a sense, the girl in this situation is being used by her mate as a way of boosting his own image. He believes that women should look a

Your weight in kilograms

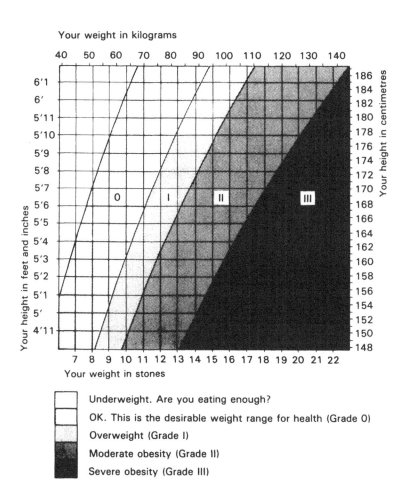

Underweight. Are you eating enough?
OK. This is the desirable weight range for health (Grade 0)
Overweight (Grade I)
Moderate obesity (Grade II)
Severe obesity (Grade III)

Source: Health Education Authority, London
Figure 3 Weight chart

95

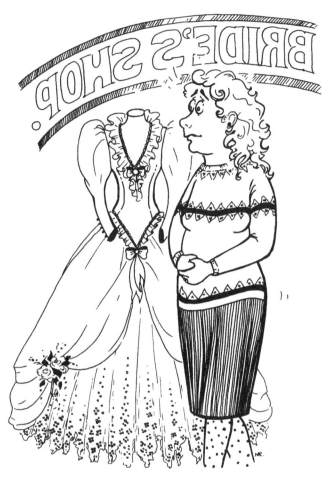

'Are you sure this is the size I ordered?'

certain way, and while he is himself happy to be with her, he would feel better if she could help him to project the right image. Whether the weight loss is necessary for the woman's health or not, nothing can be more demoralizing for the would-be dieter than the thought that a loved one will find them fully acceptable only when they have lost weight, and hence changed in shape.

So if you are about to embark on a slimming diet, one of the questions you need to ask yourself is 'Who am I doing it for?' If indeed you are doing it for someone else, how worthy are that person's motives? If he or she cannot accept you for who you are, is this really your problem or is it theirs?

Other people apart, it is important to consider what being overweight or being slim means to you personally. Most people will answer that of course they want to be slim; that slimness is their ideal, whereas being overweight has no advantages whatsoever. You should try to make a list of all the advantages being slimmer would bring you – in terms of your health, your personal life, and your work life. Make sure that you are being realistic here and not over-valuing the advantages of slimness. Make another list of all the possible advantages of being fat. This may seem like a strange thing to do, but for many people largeness does appear to have advantages. For example, there are men, and women, who feel that being large gives them a kind of presence and therefore a power in relation to other people that they would not have if they were slim and more fragile or insubstantial to look at.

It may be helpful to you at this stage to do an exercise similar to that suggested by Susie Orbach in her book *Fat is a Feminist Issue*.[1] The exercise is meant for a group of women to explore together, but male or female, you might like to try it on your own, or with a friend. The exercise involves imagining yourself at a party, very fat. You get comfortable, and shut your eyes, and imagine your surroundings. You are to consider what kind of party it is, what you are doing, how you are dressed and how you feel about your clothes. Are you standing, sitting, talking to people? Who is making the first moves? You are asked to consider what 'messages' the fat is giving to other people about you, and whether being fat in this situation helps you in any way. You are then asked to repeat the exercise while imagining yourself very thin and to consider any ways in which the experience of being thin might have disadvantages, or be frightening to you. You might want to repeat this exercise while imagining yourself in a variety of situations: with friends, at work, asking a friend or colleague to do something for you, or trying to set up a new venture.

If, as a result of the exercise, you discover for example that your size does in some way have a protective role, this does not mean that you should not diet. It does mean that if you do decide to go on a diet, you will have to be prepared for changes in your feelings about yourself as you get slimmer and have some alternative strategies for dealing with problems that your fat seemed to be shielding you from. You may, for example, want to go on a course to learn to become more assertive, so that you can say 'no' to people or become better at getting other people to do the things you want them to do.

Another factor you will want to take into account when deciding whether or not to go on a diet is how successful you have been at dieting in the past, and whether or not you believe that you could lose weight by dieting now. You might like to try answering the following questions:

1 If you went on a diet tomorrow do you think you would achieve your target weight? (Remember that you can take as long as you need given that a weight loss of a half a pound to a pound a week is reasonable.)
   (a) *Yes, definitely*   (b) *Possibly*
   (c) *No, definitely not*

2 How confident are you that if you went on a diet you would be able to resist eating too much on social occasions?
   (a) *Very confident*   (b) *Quite confident*
   (c) *Not confident at all*

3 How confident are you that if you went on a diet you would be able to resist eating too much on a normal day as far as your work or social life are concerned?
   (a) *Very confident*   (b) *Quite confident*
   (c) *Not confident at all*

4 How confident are you that if you went on a diet you would be able to resist eating too much when you are feeling upset?
   (a) *Very confident*   (b) *Quite confident*
   (c) *Not confident at all*

HOW CONFIDENT ARE YOU THAT YOU COULD LOSE WEIGHT ON A DIET?

Circle the letters in the following boxes which correspond to your answers to the questions above.

1   a   b   c
2   a   b   c
3   a   b   c
4   a   b   c

If your answers were mostly (a)s, you have a definite initial advantage as confidence in the ability to diet has been pointed to as one of the predictors of diet success. Are you sure that you are not being over-confident and overlooking some of the problems that are bound to arise?

If your answers were mainly (a)s and (b)s with perhaps one (c), you may stand a good chance of getting off to a good start if only because you have begun to pinpoint where some of the problem areas might be and can therefore develop some strategies for dealing with them.

If your answers were mainly (c)s, the way you are thinking about diet will put you at a disadvantage as every setback will come as evidence to you that dieting is not for you. This may indeed be true. Either way, you should not try to diet if you feel destined to fail. Thinking in this way, you are more likely to interpret even small successes as yet another failure. Perhaps your answers are based on past experience with diet failures. The message I have tried to convey in the preceding chapters is that, while in theory it is possible for everyone to lose weight, most people fail to do so. This is not because fat people or dieters are different psychologically from thin people and people who do not need to diet. Eating habits are individual and do not distinguish fat people from thin people, and old habits are difficult to change whoever you are. Moreover, dieting produces its own problems which most of us are ill prepared for. Some people fail because they have inadequate information, some fail because their style of eating makes long-term change difficult, and others fail because they are unaware of or unable to deal with an unhelpful situation at home or at work.

You may be able to re-examine your own experience in the light of the information given in the preceding chapters. You may decide that dieting is not for you; alternatively, you may decide that you would like to try, in the knowledge that it is possible to construe dieting and weight loss in many different ways.

If your confidence in your ability to diet successfully is low, ask yourself whether there is a reason why trying to change the way you eat would be particularly difficult for you at this moment: changes in your personal life such as marriage, separation from a loved one, or even a house move can be extremely stressful and at times such as these it is particularly hard to change old habits and you would be advised not to try until you are in a more settled frame of mind.

If, having weighed up all the facts, you decide that you are ready to diet, you can increase your confidence in your ability to do so through learning more effective strategies for coping with the changes you will have to make.

In order to change any behaviour we must have an understanding of what that behaviour is and what factors in our lives are making us continue to behave in the same way. The rest of this chapter is designed to help you find out what kind of eating style you have and how it might make dieting difficult for you.

WHAT IS YOUR EATING STYLE?[2]

For each question, circle the letter next to the answer that best describes your eating style.

1 Do you feel like eating when you see other people eating?
   (a) *Hardly ever* (b) *Sometimes* (c) *Often* (d) *Nearly always*
2 Is food a comfort to you when you are feeling depressed?
   (a) *Hardly ever* (b) *Sometimes* (c) *Often* (d) *Nearly always*
3 Do you like to eat while watching TV or reading?
   (a) *Hardly ever* (b) *Sometimes* (c) *Often* (d) *Nearly always*
4 How often are you dieting?
   (a) *Hardly ever* (b) *Sometimes* (c) *Often* (d) *Nearly always*
5 Do you eat when you are feeling angry?
   (a) *Hardly ever* (b) *Sometimes* (c) *Often* (d) *Nearly always*
6 Do you eat less than usual when you are busy all day?
   (a) *Hardly ever* (b) *Sometimes* (c) *Often* (d) *Nearly always*
7 Do you only eat when you are hungry?
   (a) *Hardly ever* (b) *Sometimes* (c) *Usually* (d) *Nearly always*
8 Do you eat when you are excited about something nice happening?
   (a) *Hardly ever* (b) *Sometimes* (c) *Often* (d) *Nearly always*
9 Are you tempted to taste the food while you cook?
   (a) *Hardly ever* (b) *Sometimes* (c) *Often* (d) *Nearly always*
10 Do you deliberately choose low-calorie or 'slimmers' foods when you shop?
   (a) *Hardly ever* (b) *Sometimes* (c) *Often* (d) *Nearly always*
11 Do you eat something when you have an occasional cup of tea or coffee?
   (a) *Hardly ever* (b) *Sometimes* (c) *Often* (d) *Nearly always*

12 Do you feel guilty when you overeat?
(*a*) *Hardly ever* (*b*) *Sometimes* (*c*) *Often* (*d*) *Nearly always*

13 Do you eat when you are trying to work out the solution to a difficult problem?
(*a*) *Hardly ever* (*b*) *Sometimes* (*c*) *Often* (*d*) *Nearly always*

14 If you do not eat at fixed meal-times do you feel weak and ill?
(*a*) *Hardly ever* (*b*) *Sometimes* (*c*) *Often* (*d*) *Nearly always*

15 Do you eat less when you are feeling happy?
(*a*) *Hardly ever* (*b*) *Sometimes* (*c*) *Often* (*d*) *Nearly always*

16 Do you make a conscious effort to eat less than usual if you find you have put on weight?
(*a*) *Hardly ever* (*b*) *Sometimes* (*c*) *Often* (*d*) *Nearly always*

17 When on holiday do you gain weight if you stay in a good hotel where all your meals are provided?
(*a*) *Hardly ever* (*b*) *Sometimes* (*c*) *Often* (*d*) *Nearly always*

18 Do you keep your food intake within certain calorie limits each day?
(*a*) *Hardly ever* (*b*) *Sometimes* (*c*) *Often* (*d*) *Nearly always*

19 Do you have all your meals and snacks at fixed times every day?
(*a*) *Hardly ever* (*b*) *Sometimes* (*c*) *Often* (*d*) *Nearly always*

20 Do you eat when you are feeling bored or have nothing to do?
(*a*) *Hardly ever* (*b*) *Sometimes* (*c*) *Often* (*d*) *Nearly always*

21 If you miss a meal do you feel very hungry?
(*a*) *Hardly ever* (*b*) *Sometimes* (*c*) *Often* (*d*) *Nearly always*

22 Do you eat less when someone has upset you?
(*a*) *Hardly ever* (*b*) *Sometimes* (*c*) *Often* (*d*) *Nearly always*

23 After a meal do you 'pick' at food in the serving dishes until they are cleared away?
(*a*) *Hardly ever* (*b*) *Sometimes* (*c*) *Often* (*d*) *Nearly always*

24 Do you count calories?
(*a*) *Hardly ever* (*b*) *Sometimes* (*c*) *Often* (*d*) *Nearly always*

25 Does the smell of good food (for example fresh bread) tempt you to eat something?
(*a*) *Hardly ever* (*b*) *Sometimes* (*c*) *Often* (*d*) *Nearly always*

26 Do you spend time reading magazines and books about food and diet?
(*a*) *Hardly ever* (*b*) *Sometimes* (*c*) *Often* (*d*) *Very often*

27 Do you eat when you are feeling anxious about something?
    (a) *Hardly ever* (b) *Sometimes* (c) *Often* (d) *Nearly always*
28 Do you think about dieting?
    (a) *Hardly ever* (b) *Sometimes* (c) *Often* (d) *Nearly always*
29 Do you suffer pangs of hunger when you eat less than
    usual?
    (a) *Hardly ever* (b) *Sometimes* (c) *Often* (d) *Nearly always*
30 Are you tempted to buy snacks you hadn't planned to buy
    when you see them at the supermarket?
    (a) *Hardly ever* (b) *Sometimes* (c) *Often* (d) *Nearly always*
31 Do you give a great deal of thought to what you eat?
    (a) *Hardly ever* (b) *Sometimes* (c) *Often* (d) *Nearly always*
32 Do you eat to keep friends or family company?
    (a) *Hardly ever* (b) *Sometimes* (c) *Often* (d) *Very often*
33 Do you eat when you are feeling lonely?
    (a) *Hardly ever* (b) *Sometimes* (c) *Often* (d) *Very often*
34 Do you eat dessert even if you are not hungry?
    (a) *Hardly ever* (b) *Sometimes* (c) *Often* (d) *Very often*
35 Do you eat when you are feeling irritable or cross?
    (a) *Hardly ever* (b) *Sometimes* (c) *Often* (d) *Very often*
36 Do you avoid eating certain foods because they are
    fattening?
    (a) *Hardly ever* (b) *Sometimes* (c) *Often* (d) *Nearly always*
37 Do you eat more when you drink alcohol?
    (a) *Hardly ever* (b) *Sometimes* (c) *Often* (d) *Nearly always*
38 Do you eat when you feel you have failed in some way?
    (a) *Hardly ever* (b) *Sometimes* (c) *Often* (d) *Nearly always*
39 When people offer you tasty-looking snacks do you accept
    even if you have just eaten?
    (a) *Hardly ever* (b) *Sometimes* (c) *Often* (d) *Nearly always*
40 How often do you weigh yourself?
    (a) *Less than once a month* (b) *At least once a month*
    (c) *Once a week or more* (d) *At least once a day*
41 If you know that you will be having a big meal in the
    evening which of the following best describes the way you
    eat in the day:
    (a) *You plan to eat less beforehand but find yourself eating
    more than usual*
    (b) *You plan to eat less in preparation but end up eating
    the same as usual*

(c) *You stick to a plan of eating less the day before*

(d) *You eat whatever you fancy without thinking about it*

42 On the whole do you eat very little when with other people but a lot when you are alone?

(a) *Hardly ever* (b) *Sometimes* (c) *Often* (d) *Nearly always*

43 If you have eaten a large meal: do you

(a) *Cut down what you eat the next day*

(b) *Eat normally the next day without thinking about it*

(c) *Intend to cut down the next day but find yourself eating the same as usual*

(d) *Try to eat less the next day but find yourself eating even more than usual and carrying on in this way for the rest of the day*

Scoring the questionnaire

Most of the questions are scored 0 for an (a) response, 1 for a (b) response, 2 for a (c), and 3 for a (d). However, there are some exceptions. The grids shown on the following pages have been arranged so that all the circles in the first column score nought, all the circles in the second column score 1, all the circles in the third column score 2, and all the circles in the fourth column score 3. Circle your answers to the relevant questions on the grids. Then find your total scores.

Here is an example of how to score some imaginary questions:

Question numbers	Scores 0	1	2	3
1	a	b	©c	d
2	a	ⓑb	c	d
3	b	c	ⓓd	a
4	ⓐa	b	c	d
Totals	0	1	4	0

This person's total score to these four questions is 5.

Are you an external eater?

Add up your scores to questions 1, 3, 6, 7, 9, 11, 17, 19, 23, 25, 30, 32, 34, and 39.

Question numbers	Scores 0	1	2	3
1	a	b	c	d
3	a	b	c	d
6	a	b	c	d
7	d	c	b	a
9	a	b	c	d
11	a	b	c	d
17	a	b	c	d
19	a	b	c	d
23	a	b	c	d
25	a	b	c	d
30	a	b	c	d
32	a	b	c	d
34	a	b	c	d
39	a	b	c	d

Totals

The maximum score is 42. Anything above 22 suggests that you have at least a tendency to eat in response to external cues such as the time of day or the sight or smell of food. The higher your score the more often you eat in response to external cues. You are more likely to eat food when it is just there, as for example at the end of a meal before the plates have been cleared, or when someone offers you something delicious to eat. We are all inclined to eat more when food is tasty or simply available (see Chapter 4), so do not feel to blame if this is something that makes unplanned eating a particular problem for you when you are trying to diet. If you score 14 or less, then bravo! If you need to diet, you are at a great advantage in today's society where food is all around us and all too easily and quickly available. Either you are someone who eats mainly in response to internal, perhaps physiological cues (see also 'Does hunger drive you?', p. 107), or perhaps you have very strong self-control and are skilled at reorganizing your environment so that food cues have become less salient for you.

Do your emotions make you eat?

Add up your scores to questions 2, 5, 7, 8, 13, 15, 20, 22, 27, 33, 35, and 38.

Question numbers	Scores 0	1	2	3
2	a	b	c	d
5	a	b	c	d
7	d	c	b	a
8	a	b	c	d
13	a	b	c	d
15	a	b	c	d
20	a	b	c	d
22	d	c	b	a
27	a	b	c	d
33	a	b	c	d
35	a	b	c	d
38	a	b	c	d

Totals

There are twelve questions, so the maximum score is 36. The higher your score, the more inclined you are to eat in response to emotions or to being under stress. This is likely to be a habit established long ago, and is a killer as far as diet attempts are concerned. However, there is no evidence that eating actually makes people any less cross, less miserable, or more relaxed. So you may be able to find alternative, more helpful ways of dealing with your feelings.

Are you a restrained eater?

Add up your scores to questions 4, 10, 12, 16, 18, 24, 26, 28, 31, 36, 37, 40, 41, 42, and 43.

Question numbers	Scores 0	1	2	3
4	a	b	c	d
10	a	b	c	d
12	a	b	c	d
16	a	b	c	d
18	a	b	c	d
24	a	b	c	d
26	a	b	c	d
28	a	b	c	d
31	a	b	c	d
36	a	b	c	d
37	a	b	c	d
40	a	b	c	d
41	d	c	b	a
42	a	b	c	d
43	b	a	c	d

Totals

The maximum score is 45. A score above 26 or thereabouts would suggest that you are a restrained eater, while a score of 18 or less would suggest that you are an unrestrained eater. At the extreme ends of the scale, unrestrained eaters worry little about their weight and give little thought to food and dieting, whereas restrained eaters think about food and dieting a great deal, are constantly watching their weight, and may be vulnerable to having their restraint broken when under stress, when they are in a situation where they find themselves eating more than they would like, or when they drink alcohol. There may be some restrained eaters who have very good control, and rarely have a problem with overeating or with feeling guilty and eating even more if they should happen to overeat. There is perhaps a degree of restraint, however, that is too stringent for some people, causing a great number of problems should they need to diet. If you are a restrained eater, pay particular attention to your answers to questions 12, 37, 41, 42, and 43. If you scored mostly 3's on these questions you may need to reassess your attitude to food and eating especially if you are overweight and need to diet. You may find that you also have high scores on questions relating to emotional eating. The groups of questions are not necessarily mutually exclusive, as it is quite possible for example for emotions to have a disinhibiting effect on the normal carefulness of a restrained eater. Chapter 10 discusses ideas that some people find useful for coping with problems inherent in an emotional or restrained eating style.

Does hunger drive you?

Questions 7, 14, 21, 29, and 34 relate to this.

Question numbers	Scores 0	1	2	3
7	d	c	b	a
14	a	b	c	d
21	a	b	c	d
29	a	b	c	d
34	d	c	b	a

Totals

If you scored mainly 3's you may be very responsive to internal hunger signals and good at differentiating between internal signals and other, social or psychological signals. However, as discussed in Chapter 4, there is a great deal of doubt as to what is meant by the concept of hunger. It is possible to experience what we believe is hunger in response to all kinds of signals not necessarily related to actual deprivation.

One example of this that comes to mind is of a lady I met some years ago who had several stones in weight to lose. She had never tried dieting before, and had few preconceived ideas about what this would mean to her. During the first few weeks of her dieting attempt she began to feel extremely hungry and claimed that her intense hunger was the only possible reason she could have for wanting to break the diet. She began to keep records of what she was eating and of the situations in which she felt especially hungry. Gradually, it dawned on her that her greatest times of hunger were when she was worried about her sister who had a chronic disease needing repeated admissions to hospital, when her two young sons were playing her up, and whenever she had a disagreement with her very chauvinistic boss! One day, after she had lost a considerable amount of weight, she said,

I'm just beginning to see what the problem was before. I thought that I was hungry, but what was really happening was that I was eating all day long. Whenever anything upsetting happened, I just went on eating, and I simply didn't notice how I was feeling. Then when I had to cut down because of the diet, I realized: I was so busy worrying about and looking after everyone else; with no one to be nice to me except me, I just had to eat all the time. Now I'm having to find other ways of coping with my problems.

KEEPING A RECORD

Keeping a record of what you eat and in what circumstances is a very good way of assessing the situation before deciding to go on a diet. Most people find it very difficult at first to monitor what they eat without actually eating less. However, this does not really matter as it is not necessarily the amount that you are eating that is important as much as the style in which you eat it. Anyone can decide to go on a diet and can aim to follow a particular food plan or diet sheet or to cut out certain foods. Just as essential, however, as eating less or differently is changing the way you eat. Watching the weight is not nearly as important an element in the long run as eating habits. Given that 'hunger' is such an elusive construct and influenced more by our external world, our thoughts, and even our feelings than by our internal workings, losing weight for most people means changing habits and learning new attitudes. Keeping a record of the situations in which you eat can help to establish aspects of your eating behaviour that you may want to change in order to help you learn new habits.

There are many different ways of keeping records. One way of doing it is to have a new page of a notebook for each day, divided into columns. In the columns you may want to record what you ate and the time of day; what goes into the other columns may depend on what, on the basis of your experience, or perhaps of filling in the questionnaires in this chapter, you think your main difficulties might be. As a guide you may like to start with the format suggested in Table 2. This is a format typically used by people who are considering changing some aspect of their behaviour and who, in order to be able to devise a plan, need some idea of what the problems are, and how they are affected by day-to-day events. Once you have collected

Table 2 Monitoring your eating habits

Time	What do you eat?	Where?	Who with?	Doing what?	What happened just before?	Mood?

this kind of information for a week or two, it becomes possible to identify patterns in your eating.

The remaining chapters are designed to help you identify targets for change and cope with the inevitable problems that arise when people try to change the way they eat in particular and the way they behave in general.

Chapter Nine

COPING WITH A DIET 2: PLANNING FOR CHANGE

Long-term dieting success is not achieved merely by an act of will. Determination to succeed can have a place in a diet plan as has the dieter's belief that come what may, they will overcome all obstacles in their way. In practice, however, long-term success also depends on a combination of knowing what to do with both a readiness to recognize difficulties and the ability to plan ahead for change.

ADJUSTING YOUR EXPECTATIONS

Many diet attempts are dogged by the problem of dieters having unreasonable expectations both of themselves and of the diet. One of the most important aspects of dieting is the question of how well people expect to do and how quickly. You should not expect to lose more than two pounds a week for the first two weeks and a pound a week after that. If you lose more, consider it a bonus, but remember that a weight loss of more than two pounds a week could mean that you are losing lean tissue in addition to fat (see p. 71). If you lose less, do not be discouraged. A weight loss of half a pound a week over several weeks is better than nothing at all. Needless to say, weight losses such as these will not register on the scales which most of us have in our homes except very crudely. Frequent weighing is unhelpful, because one's weight may fluctuate during the day and from day to day by several pounds. Therefore it is a good idea to weigh no more than once a week (remembering to weigh in at the same time of day wearing the same clothes each time!). Some people find it helpful to keep a chart or at least to write down their weight at the end of every week. Some weeks on a diet one's weight remains steady or might even go up a pound or two if you just happen to have a big meal the night before. Keeping a record allows one to check that the general trend is down even if there are some weeks (entirely normal) where weight has stayed the same or gone up.

Another important aspect of dieting success of course is the level of knowledge dieters have about nutrition and how to diet. If you plan to lose more than a few pounds you should first consult your doctor. This is partly because you should check on your fitness to diet and/or take more exercise, and partly so that you can get information about the nutritional aspects of dieting. Your doctor may have a standard diet sheet or be able to refer you for a consultation with a dietitian who will be able to advise you in line with current guidelines for healthy eating and dieting.

DEVISING A PLAN

Before we can change any aspect of our behaviour we have to know exactly what it is we want to change. It is not enough simply to say to oneself 'I must eat less' or 'I must never eat another cake'. If you have read the questionnaires in Chapter 8 and in particular if you have been able to keep a record of your eating habits for one or two weeks, you may have begun to notice patterns in the way you eat. These patterns may relate to a particular time of day, or to specific situations, or they may relate strongly to your experiencing one or more moods or emotions.

Based on what you have learned from these patterns or from filling in the eating habits questionnaire, you should be able to make a list of all the general problem areas you would like to tackle. For example you may wish to snack less when alone, cut down on sweet foods, or eat less when offered food by workmates or friends. For each general behaviour you would like to change there are a number of specific practical changes you could make. For example, in order to snack less when alone you might learn to exchange high-calorie snacks for low-calorie ones, find something else to do instead, practise halving the number of snacks, or practise not snacking at particular times of the day. Any one of these practical strategies could serve as a target for change as part of your diet plan.

Only you can know which particular strategy will be right for you. In order to choose a target for change you need to list all the possible solutions and consider the advantages and disadvantages of each one. It is also extremely important not to set out to achieve something that you know from past experience is impossible for you. Each target should be something that you will have to concentrate on but not so difficult that you are bound to fail from the start. Consider the following imaginary example.

Mrs A has been on a reducing diet but is not losing weight. She decides to keep an eating diary for two weeks. At the end of that time she notes that she eats three reasonably well-balanced meals in the day and cuts out extra bread and butter and sweet puddings. However, her record tells her that she also consumes several extra bits during the day – biscuits, the remains of food offered to visitors – and particularly during the evening, in front of the TV.

She considers the following possible solutions:

1 Decide never to eat another biscuit again.
2 Allow herself two biscuits a day and replace others with small pieces of fruit or vegetable.
3 Stop watching TV and go to bed early.
4 Decide not to have any biscuits in the house.

We could consider two possible endings to the story.

Ending 1. The first solution is the most tempting and Mrs A decides to try it this way. Delighted with her resolution, she happily resists eating biscuits all day for the next day. She thinks off and on how 'good' she is being and is totally uninterested in the idea of a biscuit even when she is offered one. The next day, biscuits seem a little more tempting. She finds herself thinking off and on about how nice it would be to have just one biscuit. Her thoughts about biscuits become mixed with thoughts like 'I really must stop thinking about food', 'I've got no control'. Then later, 'Oh I'll never do it, I might as well have one', until finally she takes a biscuit. Needless to say she does not enjoy eating the biscuit and, furious with herself, she thinks, 'I've failed again; I can never stick to a diet'. Very soon she gives up the whole attempt in despair.

The problem with this attempt is that Mrs A makes herself a promise which she knows from past experience of liking biscuits she will never be able to keep. Therefore one slip-up means that she has 'broken' the whole diet. Moreover, the self-recriminations which follow the failure of this attempt can only make matters worse. Notice also how, in this example, what people feel and think about themselves can influence what they do. The importance of thoughts in relation to trying to change behaviour will be discussed in more detail in Chapter 10.

> **Ending 2.** Mrs A is tempted to try solution 1 but knows from past experience that she would not be able to keep such a promise and that if she tried and failed she would feel bad and risk jeopardizing the success of the entire diet. The second solution is feasible but would require some planning in advance to have the right foods available and avoid impulse eating. The third solution would be fine but would not work for more than a few days. The last solution would certainly remove temptation but is not entirely within Mrs A's control as she has grown-up children and a lodger all of whom buy in their own favourite foods occasionally.
>
> Therefore solution 2 becomes her initial target for change. She decides on the specific strategy of allowing herself one or two biscuits per day and keeping low-calorie snacks (fruit, vegetables) in the 'fridge for the times when she wants something more. Every day that she succeeds with her plan she gives herself a mental pat on the back. On the days that she eats more than one or two biscuits she tells herself, 'It took me a long time to learn my old eating habits. It may take me some time to change them, but one slip-up does not mean the end of the diet.'

This particular solution may not work for everyone. Yet there are some simple messages intended in this story that could be useful to anyone wishing to change an old habit. These are:

1 Set yourself a target that you can achieve. You can move on to trying something more difficult later on. Make it a behaviour target, a specific target.
2 If the target you have set yourself does not work, do not consider yourself a failure, but try to work out why. Were you being too ambitious?
3 If the solution does work, do not just take the success for granted, but give yourself the credit for a job well done.

LEARNING TO REWARD YOURSELF WITHOUT FOOD

Weight loss takes time, the rewards are slow in coming, and most people give up before they have had sight of the end. You may have promised yourself a holiday, a new wardrobe; but you rarely get to the stage where you feel you have deserved the prize. Therefore the immediate enjoyment you get from food has far more influence on what happens than the future possibility of being slim. It is not uncommon for dieters to reward themselves for 'good' behaviour with some of the very foods they have been trying so hard to avoid. Because weight loss in itself is rewarding for dieters, some slimming clubs donate a small prize to the person who has lost the most weight each week. However, this is not a good idea for two reasons: first, different individuals need to eat different amounts to keep them at the same weight and they lose weight at different rates; and second, reward for eating habit change works better than reward for weight loss. Moreover, people who are able to reward themselves in some way do much better in weight-reduction programmes than people whose rewards come from a therapist.

The alternative to rewarding yourself with food, or to rewarding yourself only when you have lost weight, is to rearrange things so that you get frequent rewards for eating less; and instead of relying for praise or reward on someone else, you should plan to do it for yourself.

The idea of rewarding oneself may seem a little strange to some people who are not accustomed to patting themselves on the back. If you consider, however, that you may have no hesitation about making yourself a hot drink on a cold day or pouring yourself a whisky after a stressful time, then telling yourself that you have done a good job in the face of adversity is surely no different?

Whenever you choose a target, you should choose a reward to go with it. This could be something you like doing, such as watching an hour's TV, reading a magazine, telephoning a friend; or something small that you can buy for yourself: a special soap, a bottle of after-shave, a paperback novel. Alternatively you could reward yourself with small sums of money or with 'points' to be saved up towards a grand long-term reward – a new outfit, an outing to the theatre, a weekend away. Of course, taste is a very individual matter, and your own reward 'menu' shown below is just an example of the kind of list you might want to draw up for yourself:

REWARD 'MENU'

Short-term Rewards

Things to do

Telephone a friend
Take a long bath
Read a good book
Watch an hour's TV
Take a walk
Transfer 'tokens' (buttons, marbles) from one jar to another, each
token to represent a sum of money to be put towards long-term
reward

Things to buy

A magazine
After-shave
Flowers
Toiletries
A new pen
Put money in a jar

Long-term Rewards

(Saved up from 'short-term rewards')
A holiday
A visit to the theatre
New clothes

Each time you achieve your target, reward yourself immediately.
The whole point of an immediate reward is so that you learn to pair
eating differently with something pleasant rather than with a feeling
of deprivation. Of course, as it is you who are giving the rewards,
you will say that the situation is false: that you could have these
things anyway. But the point of the exercise is not so much to
acquire things you could not otherwise have as to acknowledge to
yourself that you have done well.

What about punishment?

Very often when psychologists talk about how to encourage behaviour change they are asked about punishment. For example, people ask about aversion therapy to stop them eating particular foods such as cakes or chocolate. In general, therapies which include some kind of punishment are not as effective as those in which rewards play a major part in helping people to change their behaviour. Some researchers have claimed success in using aversion therapies (where something nasty like an electric shock or the thought of being sick is paired with the sight of favourite cakes or chocolates); but while these therapies might stop people from eating specific food items, the effects do not necessarily last, or extend to other kinds of food. More importantly, punishment teaches people what not to do but does not teach them what to do instead. This is why punishments such as the occasional slap work with children as long as there is plenty of opportunity for them to learn the rewards of being good; but they do not work if they are the only way of stopping children from being naughty.

Unfortunately, people on diets have a tendency to punish themselves for not losing weight if only by the things they say to themselves. Many are prepared without question to accept criticism, and return week after week to their slimming club or doctor to be chastised for not losing weight. However, the practice of some slimming club leaders of singling out unsuccessful losers can be particularly unhelpful. Being singled out if only to discuss difficulties can at best embarrass and at worst put to shame the unsuccessful dieter. Club leaders and professionals need to learn that chastisement is belittling and unhelpful, and dieters must learn not to invite or encourage it.

ALTERING YOUR SURROUNDINGS TO MAKE FOOD LESS IMPORTANT

The first behaviour therapy programmes made the assumption that overweight people eat differently from thin people and respond more readily to external cues like the sight of food. Many slimming programmes have been written based on these ideas. They are called 'self-control' programmes because their aim is to teach people to control both the way in which they eat (how fast, and so on) and the amount of food available around them. An American psychologist, Richard Stuart, became famous for the success he had with a programme which he later published together with Barbara Davis in a detailed manual entitled *Slim Chance in a Fat World*.[1] Many of the ideas have been successfully incorporated into the Weight Watchers programmes. We now know that the assumption that fat people eat differently from thin people is on the whole untrue. People have their own individual eating styles and both fat and thin people can be 'external' eaters. Nevertheless the so-called 'self-control' programmes do work for many people, presumably because they offer practical ideas about controlling the amount of food they eat.

If you tend towards being an external eater, some of the following suggestions might help you to plan for change.

Place

If you are someone who eats in several rooms in the house, or wanders around idly munching, it may be helpful to you to decide to eat in one place only, preferably sitting down, at a table. Perhaps you eat while watching the TV or reading a book. The more able you are to make eating a 'pure' experience, the less inclined you will be to eat just out of habit, because that is usually what you do when the TV is on, while you are reading, or because you happen to see food lying around. Some people have suggested that you are very rigid about this, eating always in the same place. This means for example that if you are in the lounge watching the TV and you fancy a piece of cheese you have to go to the kitchen, eat, and return to the TV when you have finished. If you want another piece you have to go back, cut another piece, eat it there, and return to the TV again; but the idea is not to bring the whole cheese into the TV room with you. Another technique is to eat everything with a knife and fork, on a plate; this goes for anything – apples, even chocolate. The reasoning behind this is that you therefore restrict the surroundings in which you eat, which may as a consequence help you to eat less, particularly of snack food.

Eating when you see food

Do you find it hard to resist eating when you see food? For example you may eat because other people are eating, or polish off leftovers ('it's not worth leaving that little bit'). You might try keeping snack foods in opaque containers out of impulse range in a cupboard;

getting the family to prepare and fetch their own snacks; having low-calorie snacks available to eat while other people are nibbling. If you find it hard to resist leftover food, practise throwing it away. This is something that many of us find very difficult; but there is no point in leaving it sitting in the 'fridge to tempt you if you are going to spend half an hour soul-searching and end up eating it anyway. It is quite reasonable to exercise control by making leftover food unavailable in the waste-bin. Perhaps at a later stage in your programme you will be better able to resist food that is on show but if you cannot at first, there is no point in struggling. Throwing away leftover food is no more wasteful than eating it yourself if you have no need for it, in which case it can do a great deal of harm to you and your self-esteem and no good whatsoever to the starving masses.

Another way of decreasing contact with food is to keep problematic food out of the house if possible or to avoid situations where you might buy it out of habit. An obvious example is to shop with a list, so as to avoid buying calorific treats or special offers at the supermarket checkout. You might make it a target not to buy biscuits or snack foods 'for the children' or 'in case we have visitors' (will there really be any left for the visitors?). If you cannot walk past the cake shop or the confectioner's without going in, try walking round the shops or home from work in a different direction.

Thoughts about food

Thoughts about food can cause us to eat just as much as the sight of food. An advertisement on the TV, a picture in a magazine, or the thought of food in a bored moment can send us straight to the kitchen or a snack bar. Of course if you are trying to diet, thoughts about food are more likely to occur. Try to decide whether you are really hungry or not. This is not easy, but you may perhaps have just eaten; you may be particularly vulnerable to thinking about food when bored or miserable or perhaps just seeing and thinking about food makes you want it. If you have decided that you have no reason for physical hunger, you might try distracting yourself from the thought of food by doing something else, perhaps taking some exercise.

IS THE WAY YOU EAT A PROBLEM?

If you eat very fast, sometimes perhaps without realizing how much you have eaten, it may help to take some practical steps to alter the way you eat. You could try eating more slowly. You could practise chewing your food more slowly, keeping the food in your mouth for longer intervals before swallowing. In order to slow the pace of eating even further, you might try pausing between mouthfuls, putting your knife and fork down while you swallow, and picking them up again when your mouth is empty. You might practise making the intervals between mouthfuls longer by counting to a higher number each time.

Some of these techniques have been described countless times before and many run the risk of offending people perhaps to the point of insult by virtue of their very simplicity. Dieters might be excused for doubting that they could offer any solution to a complex diet problem. Certainly they are not all relevant to every dieter; but where they are relevant to a particular problem, they may be worth a try, as sometimes the most simple solutions are very effective. The purpose of each one is to change a very well-established habit, and old habits are often the unadaptive bricks our problems are built with.

The key to success is to tackle problems gradually. If on the basis of the questionnaires you filled in and the records you have kept you were able to identify some targets for change, you should not try to change everything at once. Changing old habits takes time. Before you can say that a habit has changed, you will have had several false starts: you will simply have forgotten your intentions on some occasions; you will have tried to do things differently only to be foiled by a friend (offering you food, making you a cake), by the weather (you prepared a low-calorie, health food picnic but it rained and everyone went to the hamburger restaurant), and countless other unexpected events created by other people, your environment, or you yourself. It is better to succeed with changing one small habit than to fail at an attempt to change everything at once.

It is important to keep a record of your progress, every day if possible. If putting pen to paper seems too much like hard work, do bear in mind that many of us when we are trying to change old habits remember only our failures and forget the times when things went well. Writing things down will underline your successes and

119

Table 3 Record of progress with weekly targets

Target for this week . . .

Day	Number of times I had the opportunity to practise	Number of times I succeeded	What made it easier	What made it harder	I rewarded myself with

help you to work out what to do when things go wrong. Table 3 gives an example of the kind of record you might keep.

INCREASING EXERCISE

You can plan to take more exercise in the same way as you can plan to eat differently. There is no need to start running marathons. You might simply find a way gradually to increase the amount of exercise you do already. For example you might practise using the stairs more often instead of the lift or the escalator; or getting off the bus one or two stops earlier on the way to work. You could keep a record of these activities just as you do food-related targets, and plan to award yourself points for every time you achieve a particular target or a reward for achieving a particular increase over, say, one or two weeks.

DEALING WITH FAMILY AND FRIENDS

Another important way of ensuring that you control the amount and type of food in your environment is through family and friends.

People around us have a strong if subtle effect on what we do and think. There is always someone who is giving praise, criticism, and advice. Let us consider some of the effects of other people on what we eat.

People offer food on social occasions. Accepting or not accepting the food they offer may be taken as a sign of how polite we are. The attitude of different people in this respect varies between groups from one extreme of total indifference to the other extreme of seeing food and whether it is offered or accepted as a sign of how much people like each other. People offer food as a reward: for example as a special meal for a birthday treat, to cheer someone up if they are feeling miserable; a gift of chocolates to say 'thank you' or 'congratulations'. For a mother, cooking meals may be one of her most important jobs and the family may be upset if she tries to change what she cooks. No doubt, every person who reads this book will be able to think of other ways in which food figures in the key relationships in their life.

As well as the general part food plays in your life, there is the particular effect on you of what people say about food, or about your attempts to diet.

Consider the emotional blackmail inherent in the remark: 'Go on, another cake (potato, biscuit, etc) won't hurt; I made it myself.' Then there is the refusal to take you seriously: 'You are OK as you are. All your/our family are fat. It wouldn't suit you to be thin.'

Perhaps more destructive is teasing: 'Another of your crazy diets? I don't know why you bother. It won't work anyway'; or criticism: 'You shouldn't be eating that.' For many people, being criticized for something tends to make them do it all the more.

Another unhelpful attitude is plain indifference. No one notices what you eat; they make no effort to avoid eating high-calorie snacks in front of you, and make no comment either to praise or criticize, whether you lose or gain weight.

Habit change is a very difficult task, and you need all the help you can muster. If you are lucky, it may be possible to get some help from family and friends. Here are some suggestions you might try.

1 Inform them about your attempt to change your eating habits. Make it clear that this is not just a fad diet, but a serious experiment in which you, the investigator, are trying to find the most permanent and satisfactory way of changing the way you eat in order to lose weight.

2 Explain that the emphasis is not on pounds or will-power but on habit change. Ask them to pay less attention to what you weigh and more attention to your gradual attempt to change what you eat.

3 Tell them you are trying to take the emphasis off food in your life. Ask them as a general rule not to offer you food; not to ask you to prepare extra snack food for them but to get it themselves.

4 Explain that criticism does not help but that you would value their praise and encouragement wherever possible: for example when you tell them that you have reached a target such as eating less of a particular food or when they notice you exchanging a high-calorie snack for a low one.

You in turn can help your family and friends to change their behaviour towards you.

Thank them whenever they praise you; and when they help to keep food at a 'low profile': for example by not offering you food or by snacking on a food that you dislike instead of eating your favourite chocolates in front of you. The more you praise a person for something that they do, the more likely they will be to do it again. Tell them about your progress; describe your weekly targets. When you achieve a target, tell them about it.

If your efforts to change the things your family and friends do and say do not work, consider why this might be. Do they think that you do not need to diet because you are not overweight? If so, then are you dieting unnecessarily? Perhaps they are overweight too and jealous of your efforts, or simply do not take them seriously.

If, in the end, you cannot gain the support of your spouse, your family, or your friends in your diet attempt, this need not be a reason to give up in despair. It is perfectly possible for people to diet successfully without this kind of help. The key then is to make sure that you treat it as a practical problem-solving exercise in which you set about learning what are the things that make dieting more or less difficult for you and determine to create an environment for yourself which will help you stage by stage to achieve what you want.

CHILDREN AND DIETS

You could use the techniques described in this chapter to help a child with his or her diet. Dieting is more complicated for children than for adults, because while you might want to stop sideways growth, you will want to ensure that the child is still growing upwards. It is difficult to estimate exactly how much a child needs in order to grow upwards but not outwards, and for any radical dietary changes it is best to obtain skilled dietary advice from a dietitian. Once you have done this, however, there is no reason why you should not apply some of the principles described above.

Diets with children are most successful in the long term when one or more of their parents have been closely involved in learning about how to keep the diet going, even to the extent of eating the same kinds of food and joining the child in making sure that he or she avoids certain items. This does not necessarily mean that the parent needs to keep to the diet alongside the child in the long term; simply supporting the child in the business of making the environment as conducive to the diet as possible and rewarding the child appropriately may be all that is needed.[2]

It goes without saying that no child can be expected to cut out foods that the rest of the family are eating, or not to eat birthday cake at a friend's party. Yet if the idea of having particular weekly targets and perhaps of keeping records of how far these are achieved is understood, it should be possible for a child over the age of 7 or 8 to exercise a certain degree of self-control. For example, the child could be taught to use the 'traffic light' system whereby foods called 'green' can be eaten freely, foods called 'orange' can be eaten in moderation, and foods called 'red' avoided if possible.[3] A weekly target might be for the child to eat fewer than four 'red' foods, or to practise saying 'no' when offered food by friends or relatives. The parent could spend time with the child at the end of every day in order to keep a daily progress chart. There is plenty of room for the use of imagination in the use of such charts. For example, coloured stickers might be used to denote the number of times the child ate a red food, or green for the number of times a green food was chosen instead. Brightly coloured stars might be used for the attainment of particular targets, such as losing a pound in weight, not snacking between certain meals, or helping to choose appropriate foods at the supermarket.

123

The use of rewards with children needs to be handled very sensitively. It is important that the rewards are not seen as bribes, to be manipulated at the whim of both parties. A list of appropriate rewards should be drawn up by parent and child together. These should either be small enough to allow their use frequently or, if the child is old enough to understand the system, achievable by the accumulation of points. Exactly which reward goes with which behaviour must be agreed with the child from the start, and preferably written down clearly, to save argument later on. It should be possible for the child to receive rewards frequently, especially at first. This means that the targets must be easy enough for the child to achieve. Rewards when they are deserved should be delivered immediately, and every time, otherwise the system loses its value, just as it does with adults. They should not be food rewards, and should not be things that are too often available at other times. Perhaps the most important point to make is that rewards which are part of a system devised to help a child gain self-control over eating and keep to a diet should not be confused with other things. It should be made clear that they are part of a special system, and whatever else happens in the child's day they cannot be won for doing other things or taken away for being naughty.

Finally, it is just as important, if not more so, to give children praise for achieving their targets as it is to reward them with things. The reward, just as it is with adults, is only a sign of their success and means nothing on its own. A 'well done', 'aren't you clever', or a hug and a kiss will in the end mean more than tangible rewards and the praise will in itself help to make the reward, and therefore the achievement, more meaningful.

WHEN YOUR EMOTIONS MAKE YOU EAT

Most of the strategies discussed in this chapter are aimed at the external eater. They make the assumption that all that is needed to keep to a diet is good environmental planning. This of course is not true, as most people who have tried dieting have found to their cost.

If you had a high score on the emotional eating section of the questionnaire in Chapter 8 you may find it very easy to diet for short periods of time and then find yourself giving up over an upset or some excitement. Perhaps you are aware that there are times when you eat but are not really hungry. Do you eat mainly when you are bored, miserable, or angry? There is a whole host of emotions that may trigger eating, but sometimes a habit of eating in response to emotions is so ingrained that it is very difficult for the person to recognize what is happening. This is where keeping a written record can help. Each time you feel like eating when you have reason to believe that you ought not to be hungry, stop and wait five minutes before eating. Try to decipher what you are feeling. Are you feeling cross about something, discouraged, or just bored? Try to write down what happens on these occasions. Once you have deciphered for yourself what is really happening, you may decide not to eat. If at worst, you do still eat on this occasion, you may be able to work out a way of reacting differently next time.

To begin with, you might try simply distracting yourself from food. Removing yourself physically from the place where food is kept, finding something else to do which would make it difficult to eat at the same time such as taking a bath, or absorbing yourself in a complicated piece of work are just some possibilities.

The key to successful change is forward planning. If you can identify the problems which make dieting difficult for you, you may be able to plan strategies for dealing with them in advance. For example, if you tend to eat when you are bored, you may need to plan ahead by taking up a new hobby or by arranging your day differently. Perhaps you eat when you feel angry. If so, is there something you could do about it which will ensure that your anger is not turned in on you, but directed outwards to whatever it was that caused it? For example, it may help for you to speak your mind to someone. Perhaps someone has taken advantage of you – for example a family member expecting you to clear up after them, someone at work expecting you to do more work than is reasonable. Decide for yourself whether you are justified in feeling the way you do and, if appropriate, be assertive about getting what you want or ensuring that people do not take advantage of you.[4]

You may not immediately be able to identify why it is that you are feeling upset. You may simply be feeling tense and 'uptight' after a difficult day at work or after a particularly awkward time with friends and relatives. In this situation active relaxation is a good first aid measure and may even help you to see a more effective way of reorganizing things the way you want them.

One way of relaxing is to do some physical exercise such as going for a walk or a swim (not necessarily very strenuous).

Alternatively, you could relax by doing some relaxation or yoga exercises. The important thing to remember about relaxation exercises is that whatever method you use, you cannot expect to be entirely relaxed the first time you try. Relaxation is a skill, like riding a bicycle or driving a car. You need to practise going through the motions in a quiet place, for perhaps half an hour a day. It is better to practise little and often than long and rarely. If you are using a tape, you should try as soon as possible to master the exercises without the tape so that the relaxation becomes something you can do for yourself rather than something which you can do only in a particular place, under particular circumstances. With most schedules it does not matter if you cannot remember the exercises in the exact order they were first presented or if you miss one or two out, as long as you can remember the ones that are of most benefit to you personally. As you become more practised you should try taking 'time out' during the day to relax. You may be able to adapt your exercises or shorten them so that there are one or two things that you can do while sitting in the office, the car, the train, or even while walking or doing household chores. You can only reap the full benefit of learning to relax when your new skill becomes something you can summon up easily, perhaps by repeating a certain phrase to yourself, conjuring up a relaxing scene, or taking a few deep breaths, breathing out very slowly each time, and relaxing as you breathe out.[5]

Chapter Ten

ALTERNATIVES TO WILL-POWER

Repeated dieting has the effect of lowering your metabolic rate each time and making you prone to putting on weight more quickly afterwards (see Chapter 6). For this reason, if you do want to diet it is vital to ensure that you have the best possible chance of succeeding. The strategies described in the preceding chapter were designed to help you to do this.

However, you would not be human if your attempts did not sometimes come to nothing or your newly learned eating habits abandon you in times of stress. This is where, for some people, their problems begin and the diet ends; but there is no need for this to happen if you are prepared.

COPING WITH RELAPSE

Sooner or later everyone who diets 'relapses', in other words returns to their old way of eating. Some people are able to put themselves back on the diet track very quickly, but for most this is the beginning of the end. Relapse is more likely to happen to dieters who have put themselves on a strict regime which is very different from their old way of eating than to dieters who are making gradual changes. The strict dieter may see the situation as one of being either 'on' the diet or 'off' the diet, with no middle path. As soon as he or she has made even one small slip, all is lost and the diet has failed. In other words, what happens to you on a diet can depend very largely on the way you feel the diet is going. On the other hand, the dieter who sees the diet as just a way to make some gradual changes can view the odd occasion when a target is not reached as unimportant.

One way to avoid relapse then is to ensure that you are realistic about the kind of diet you take on.

Once a diet or eating change is under way, however, it is important to accept that there will be times when new habits will be difficult to keep up and that the times of most difficulty cannot be overcome without some careful planning. The first step in this process is for the dieter to recognize in which situations he or she is at the most risk. 'To be forewarned is to be forearmed.' This is where careful record-keeping can help. The next step is to devise some strategies for dealing with the situations. For example, someone who has decided to avoid eating sweet sugary things might find themselves invited to a party where they know that many of the foods available will be on their list of things to avoid. One option would be to decide beforehand to eat whatever is available and return to the diet the next day. Alternatively, however, the dieter might decide that in view of the long-term changes they are attempting to make, they would prefer to find some way of not eating these foods. The principle here is not to rely on 'will-power', whatever that may be, but to exercise choice. Thinking about it beforehand can help you to decide what you will eat instead, whether to eat before you go to the party or what you will say if someone tries to press food on you.

Learning to be assertive

Most of the problems dieters come across in relation to other people can be overcome by being assertive, in other words being firm about what they want without being aggressive. Some of us (and not only dieters) have a great deal of difficulty in telling other people what we want from them or simply in saying 'no'. One way of dealing with the social problem is to telephone your host when you are invited out and tell him or her that you do not eat puddings/chips, or whatever particular foods you are trying to cut down on; alternatively you might decide just to go along and see what happens, having made the decision that you will simply say 'no' to some things. In either case you might arrive to find that the table is laden with high-calorie foods, and few alternatives. 'Oh, it won't hurt you this once,' your host might say, adding for final effect to the assembled guests, 'After all we can't be on a diet all the time, can we?' You have the option of saying 'No thank you' and going hungry or of eating food that you would prefer not to. On other occasions you may be faced with more choice but still be in the position of having to say 'no' to certain items of food. The success with which you are able to do this will depend both on how convinced you are that this is what you want and how good you are at being firm. If you hesitate this may be interpreted as indecision and your host/ess may ply you all the harder. The way you say 'no' is also important. Remarks like 'Well I'm not supposed to' or 'I shouldn't really' are invitations to people to try to persuade you that you should, and you could easily become involved in an uncomfortable discussion about whether you really need to diet or an argument about whether there are more calories in four ounces of pudding than there are in an apple.

When you really want to say 'no', say it with conviction: 'No, I won't thank you.' When your host tries to persuade you, repeat your answer and do not make excuses. If you wish to, say 'It looks very nice' or 'I'm sure it's wonderful' but stick to your guns, 'I won't, thank you'. As always when you are being assertive it helps to use a similar phrase each time you have to repeat yourself. This way, no one can get you involved in an argument. You will be better prepared if you go over the scene beforehand, either in your mind, going over the things you are going to say and preparing yourself for all the counter-arguments, or out loud, perhaps acting out the situation with a friend.

When you cannot say no

Unfortunately, many people cannot say 'no' to food, not for lack of being assertive, but because they cannot resist eating. If you are a 'restrained' eater, you may find yourself eating more when you want to eat less and the temptations available at a social gathering may break a previously firm control. Invariably, overeating on occasions such as these is followed by intense remorse and self-recrimination, which serve only to make matters worse. Alternatively, you may find that you have iron control when in the company of other people but that you go on a binge when you are at home on your own.

LEARNING TO DEAL WITH COMPULSIVE EATING

The power of our thoughts

As we have seen in earlier chapters of this book, the amount we eat is often connected with our thoughts or beliefs about the food we are eating and the effect it has on us.

Our thoughts are with us all the time. In the private conversations we have in our heads, we comment on what we are doing, plan ahead, go over things that have happened, or perhaps have imaginary conversations with other people. We all of us vary in the extent to which we can conjure up scenes for ourselves, but however imaginative or not we are, our thoughts are never mere echoes of factual events. They are coloured by the way we feel about things and therefore they in turn can make us feel better or worse.

Invariably the kinds of things we say to ourselves when we fail to do what we intended are negative. An American psychiatrist, Professor Arnold Beck, has categorized some of the negative things people say to themselves when they are depressed and has been in the forefront of new developments in a psychological therapy for depression, called 'cognitive therapy'. The therapy starts with helping people to recognize the negative things they say to themselves so that they can begin to replace the thoughts with more positive, helpful ones and start to feel better as a consequence.[1] In the case of binge eating, or of overeating when on a diet, there are some typical statements that many dieters will recognize. These often fall into similar categories. Here are some examples:

All or nothing thinking

You think in terms of black and white. Therefore if you cannot do a thing perfectly you see yourself as a total failure.

I must never eat ice-cream/ butter/bread, etc.

I'm a total failure.

I've got no self-control.

Overgeneralization
You see a single negative event as proof of general failure or interpret every instance of eating a high-calorie food as evidence of impending weight gain.

I've blown the diet now with that cake/meal, so I might as well carry on eating/give up.

I'll put on weight if I eat that.

Labelling
Instead of describing what has happened you attach a negative label to yourself.

I'm such a pig.

Why am I so pathetic/ stupid?

Should (or ought) statements
The 'conscience' in your head is continually telling you what to do and what not to do. Like a bossy parent, this only makes you feel guilty or angry.

I shouldn't have eaten that.

I should be able to stick to my diet.

Predicting the future
(Fortune-telling.) You are convinced that things will turn out badly as if the future is already fact.

I'm going to fail at dieting.

I'll never be slim.

I'll get fat.

Discounting the positive
You automatically focus on your failures, on the bad things that happen to you, and don't recognize small successes or notice the good things that happen.

So what if I lost a pound this week (I should have lost six by now), my clothes still don't fit me.

So I didn't have dessert; after what I ate yesterday I didn't need a main course either.

If you recognize any or all of these statements as the triggers or results of your own diet relapses, it might be worth examining how helpful or not they are in your diet attempts.

Looking for alternative thoughts

Try to be more aware of the things you say to yourself when things go wrong, and think about how true or reasonable they are. If a diet is proving very difficult for you, you might try keeping a record of all the times when you did not keep to your plan, and writing down the thoughts you were having at the time. Ask yourself how helpful it is to you to think in this way. Is there an alternative way for you to view the problem? How could you rephrase your comments so that you can feel positive about making further changes rather than falling into a vicious cycle of despair, further eating, and more despair?

This is not the same as suggesting that dieters use 'positive thinking'. Positive thinking can be as unhelpful as negative thinking if you are saying positive things merely as an exercise without believing them. The point of the exercise is to examine the automatic thoughts you have when you are feeling bad and learn to interpret what has happened in a more realistic way.

Consider the following example. Gail has been dieting successfully for a fortnight. She is at home alone one evening, feeling moody and irritable. She raids the biscuit tin, and then feels full of remorse. 'I shouldn't have done that,' she says to herself, 'I'll put on weight. I've got no self-control. I'll never succeed at dieting, I might as well give up altogether.' One negative thought follows another: a 'should' statement; an overgeneralization; thinking in all or nothing terms, and predicting the future. The disadvantage of thinking in this way is that Gail begins to feel even more miserable than she was before. If eating is something she tends to do when under stress, she is now more likely than she was before to return to the biscuit tin and empty it or go out to buy some more.

An alternative strategy might be for her to sit down and think about what has happened in a different way. First, she will need to examine the facts. These are: that she has been keeping successfully to her plan for two weeks (therefore she must have at least some self-control); that on this one occasion she has eaten more than she had planned to; she might also have been trying to avoid eating these particular biscuits; probably, if she does not continue to eat packets of biscuits, this 'slip' will make no difference to her weight at the next weighing. At worst she may have remained the same weight as she was previously. Where then is the evidence that she has 'no self-control', that she 'will never succeed', that she 'will put on weight'?

Second, she will need to think of some more realistic things she can say to herself which will help her not to feel so bad. For example, she might tell herself that she has done very well to keep to her diet for a fortnight without slipping. No one is perfect; anyone can make a mistake. The lesson to be learned from the episode is that she needs to find a way of coping with being fed up that does not involve eating.

None of this is easy for dieters. One of the reasons for this is that there are certain errors in thinking that all of us make so frequently that we are unaware of them. For example, 'should' or 'ought' statements are so common that we seldom stop to examine their validity. If this is something that you are aware of doing, ask yourself why *should* you be able to diet or stop yourself eating compulsively? It is natural for people to have difficulty in restricting their intake. There may be additional reasons why dieting is particularly difficult in your own circumstances: for example, you may have a hectic job which makes meal-planning difficult; a young family for whom you are continually preparing food; or perhaps you are depressed and under par, and eating is a major comfort to you.

If it is impossible for you to move away from an all-or-nothing stance with regard to dieting or eating, consider the advantages of seeing yourself as a failure or of feeling guilty. You may believe that guilt should stop you from repeating your mistakes. Unfortunately this does not happen. Feeling guilty has the disadvantage of making you feel worse, and therefore may simply cause you to eat more.

Learning to give up a restrained eating style

Another possible lesson from the example of Gail's diet attempt given above is the need to be aware of the possible effects of a restrained eating style on the tendency to overeat. A major assumption on which Gail based her tirade at herself was that biscuits are fattening. Many people who have dieted frequently make a very clear distinction between what they consider to be 'fattening' or 'non-fattening' foods, between being 'good' and being 'bad'. Hence, for example, certain foods such as bread, butter, potatoes, in addition to processed foods such as chocolate and pies, are 'bad'; whereas cottage cheese, salad, apples, natural yoghurt, crispbreads, are 'good'. The problem for people who make this kind of distinction is that their diet may become extremely restricted. To take an extreme example of a woman who has set very rigid boundaries for herself: she may have no problems as long as she can herself control the type of food she buys and eats; but even a slight transgression of her 'good'/'bad' food boundary, either as a result of being in a social situation where she cannot help eating a 'banned' food or as a result of a craving, can lead to her totally abandoning her restraint and binge eating uncontrollably.

If this kind of all-or-nothing thinking could be a problem for you, it would make sense to consider how far it is necessary entirely to exclude certain items of food from your diet. Examine the evidence for considering potatoes or bread, for example, as 'bad'. Weight for weight and calorie for calorie, how do they compare with foods you *are* prepared to eat? Even if they have more calories, how do they compare in nutritional value or in the extent to which they fill you up? Is there any real advantage in two slices of crispbread over one slice of wholemeal bread?

It may be helpful to reintroduce 'banned' foods gradually to your diet, so that you no longer have to avoid contact with them through fear. Choose one or two to start with, and test out whether by eating a little, for example, of bread, or potato, your worst fears of putting on weight or growing fat are realized.

Deprivation does not work

Compulsive eating is a fairly subjective problem in that one person's binge may be another person's snack, and one person's meal may be another's binge. Occasional overeating may be a fairly normal habit, especially for people who are dieting. However, you may have a serious problem if for several weeks and more you have been regularly alternating a strict diet attempt (or trying to purge yourself by taking laxatives or being sick) with eating very large amounts of food without being able to stop.

If compulsive eating is a major problem for you, you will need to give up active dieting altogether until you are feeling in control and your weight is stable. It is impossible both to cope with an eating problem and to lose weight at the same time, and to expect this of yourself may only lead to further trouble.

Many people who have problems with overeating have dieted

repeatedly and each time weight loss becomes more difficult (see Chapter 6). Often one of the factors keeping a binge-eating problem going is a refusal by dieters to allow themselves to eat at regular intervals. If this has happened to you, you will need to put a stop to depriving yourself and try to regularize your eating by taking three meals a day and if possible taking small planned snacks in between.

A serious dieter or compulsive eater may scoff at this idea and say, 'But if I did this I'd be like a house!' This is not necessarily true, for two reasons. First, if you are eating very little on some days and very large amounts on other days, you may on average be eating far more than if you were to eat three meals and some snacks on all the days. Second, because of the effect of dieting on metabolism, long periods of eating very little or nothing at all followed by a large uncontrolled binge may be far more fattening than a regular meal pattern. Your body becomes accustomed to doing without food, and the calories when they do arrive are more readily stored as fat. Most researchers and therapists working in the field of eating disorders will recommend a return to a regular meal pattern as the first step in dealing with a problem. Contrary to what dieters might fear, people who are able to do this do not gain weight. Try to decide beforehand when your meals and snacks are to be. The meals do not all need to be three-course affairs, although it is a good idea to avoid restricting them to salad only! For a snack you could take some clear soup, a couple of biscuits, or a piece of fruit. Try not to skip a meal just because you are busy, at work, or distracted. Gradually, as you allow yourself to eat at mealtimes, the urge to eat compulsively will recede and become easier to handle. If you find this reasoning hard to believe, you might try eating meals as an experiment. Weigh yourself at the beginning of the week, and after one week of eating regular meals and trying not to binge in addition, weigh yourself again. If your weight is the same, you will know that you *can* eat normally and not put on weight. If your weight has gone up, is it because you were binging in addition to having meals? If the answer is yes, then do not despair. Getting back to a normal pattern of eating is the first step. It will be easier for you to work out a way to give up binge eating now that you are not having to battle with deprivation as well.

Giving up compulsive eating

You can start to give up binge eating by trying not to eat in between your planned meals and snacks. Begin by tackling the time of day when this will be easiest for you. You might divide the day up into two- or three-hour periods, and make a list of the periods in order of least to most difficulty with regard to your ability to avoid eating during those times. You might treat not eating during one or more of these times as weekly targets of increasing difficulty, and in order to achieve the targets you might find it helpful to use some of the techniques described in Chapter 9. For example, you may find, on the basis of the records you have kept, that the time from when you get home from work to dinner-time is your most vulnerable: that you binge often in the evenings after dinner, and occasionally after lunch. You might begin by setting yourself the target of not eating (apart from meals) between the hours of 2.0 and 4.0 pm. When you are confident that you have achieved your target you might move on to trying to eat only a pre-planned snack after dinner, between the hours of 8.0 and 10.00 pm. Finally, you will feel ready to tackle the time of day which is usually the most difficult for you.

You should also try allowing yourself to eat without always counting calories or avoiding 'banned' foods. If you have certain 'trigger' foods which you believe cause you to overeat, consider reintroducing them gradually to your diet and work on increasing the time interval between tasting them and continuing to eat. Work on allowing yourself to go out for meals without feeling guilty or worrying about how much you are consuming.

These suggestions are not meant to imply that you should give up dieting altogether and use this as an excuse for eating as much as you like and putting on weight. The idea is that in order to give up compulsive eating and compulsive dieting it is essential to relearn to eat without excessive restraint, guilt, or self-condemnation. Only when you have once more become relaxed about eating and not eating will you be ready to consider dieting if it is necessary for you to lose weight.

FEELING GOOD ABOUT YOURSELF, FAT OR THIN

The key to successful dieting or coping with an eating problem is to feel good about yourself, come what may. This does not mean that you have to walk about with a fixed smile on your face, smugness personified; nor does it mean that you do not need to recognize your faults. It does mean that as well as being aware of faults, problems, and failures, you can forgive yourself as you would others, and at the same time recognize your assets and use them to your advantage.

If you are struggling with a diet or to cope with an eating problem, there may be some things you can do to help yourself in the meantime. One of the major disadvantages of being overweight or concerned about diet and eating is that sufferers often feel excluded from normal social activities. As we have seen (in Chapter 3) there is no doubt that people who are overweight are at a disadvantage socially; but it is all too easy for a weight or eating problem to become an excuse for not doing things in the present. How often, for example, have you said to yourself, 'When I'm slim I'll do . . .'? You may feel that changing things now is too difficult because you do not look right, because you cannot find the clothes you want, or meet the people you want to meet. Unfortunately, thinking in this way can draw you into a vicious circle of waiting until you have lost weight to do the things you want to do and not losing the weight because you feel too depressed . . .

Just as it is important to be aware of the effect of negative thoughts on your attempt to diet, it is important too to be aware of their effect on the way you feel about yourself and your size. 'I look awful', 'I feel fat', 'They'll notice how fat I am', are just some examples of thoughts which can only make you feel worse. Even if you need to slim for health reasons your negative thoughts may well be more often to do with the way you look than about the state of your health.

It is important in the first place to examine how far the things you say to yourself are a reflection of objective truth. For example, where does your weight lie according to the weight tables? Are you objectively overweight? If you are within the normal range you may need to consider how likely it is that other people see you as fat. Some dieters may feel slim one day and fat the next, depending on what clothes they wear. An observer, however, is unlikely to notice the difference.

If, however, you are overweight and it shows, or have been battling with an eating problem for some time, try to accept that this is the way you are for now. Learning to accept the way you look, problems and all, may be hard work. It means learning not to criticize yourself unreasonably and not allowing others to do so. If you criticize yourself, not only do you feel bad, but you also become less confident in doing the things you need to do, such as buying new clothes, eating in public, asserting yourself in the work-place. Learning to see yourself in a more favourable light means behaving as if you are not ashamed or embarrassed, and gradually you will find that you no longer have a problem.

You might try setting yourself targets based on learning to tackle your beliefs about the way things are for overweight people: for example, if you are overweight and feel embarrassed about eating in public, practise eating your sandwiches in front of other people, eating in the canteen at work, or eating dessert in a restaurant. If you eat compulsively, try to make eating a less shaming experience by allowing yourself to eat the foods you really want in front of other people, not hidden away as if you were committing a crime. After all, if you really want to eat, why should you feel ashamed? At each stage write down the negative thoughts you had. Try replacing them with a more realistic assessment of what was happening. For example, if you had dessert in a restaurant, how likely is it that the woman at the next table was watching what you ate? Was she thinking what a pig you were, or was she thinking about her leaking roof? Can you really guess what someone else is thinking? Do you have to care? If indeed people criticize you, deal with their criticism directly. Accept the bits that are true, and do not accept the bits that are not. For example, if you are wearing a favourite shirt in a colour that suits you and a friend says: 'That shirt is much too tight, you really shouldn't wear it,' do not necessarily rush to take it off. 'Yes, it is rather tight,' you might say, 'but the colour suits me, don't you think?'

It may also be helpful to consider what being fat means to you personally. Does it, for example, signify failure, lack of self-control? Even if your diet attempts have been a failure, does that make you a failure as a person? Is it reasonable for a person who has failed in some way to be rejected by other people? If indeed you have failed should you have to suffer further pain by rejecting yourself?

There are some dieters who operate on the belief that they cannot truly be happy until they are slim. Consider what it is that makes people happy. Is happiness really an either/or state, or are there degrees of happiness? Does happiness come from being or looking a certain way or can it come from doing things you enjoy? Is it impossible for someone who is overweight or not perfect in looks to take part in enjoyable activities? If it is important to you to be perfect, and to be perfect means slim, consider also the pressure you will be under if and when you attain your ideal weight. You will then expect yourself to be entirely happy, to have friends, recognition, love. Attractive people undoubtedly have an advantage over others but consider how far the people you care most about judge others by the way they look? How far indeed do you yourself judge a person's worth by their appearance? Do you think any the less of the people you know well who are overweight or unattractive? If you look at the people around you, is it only the most physically attractive people who have friends, lovers, family around them? If you are putting off changes in your life – making new social contacts, going for a new job – while you wait to be slim, consider making those changes now.

Removing the pressure from yourself to diet or to be slim may, at first, be an exercise in which you cannot wholeheartedly believe. With practice, however, you will find that it is possible to change old habits and beliefs until the ability to diet successfully is no longer a significant criterion by which you judge yourself.

Slimming is an exercise beset with difficulties, not least the common belief that anyone can do it. It has come to be associated with extremes of emotion suffered in private and only recently recognized. If each dieter can begin to understand a little of what happens to our bodies when we gain or lose weight, and of the effects of dieting and weight loss on the way we feel and think, then he or she may be better prepared to make a decision about whether to diet and a plan of how to go about it. Fashions are constantly changing, and the pressure to be slim is firmly a phenomenon of today. Perhaps tomorrow, large will reign again; in the meantime, however, all of us, dieters and non-dieters alike, need to separate the harsh reality of the health imperative from the fallacy of an image created by our times.

NOTES

1 A BOOK WITHOUT A PROMISE

1 'How to make light work of bubbly', *Sunday Times*, 10 May 1987, p. 31. The article reports the launch of a diet by *Debrett's Peerage*, recommending the consumption of four bottles of champagne per week. It also notes that this contradicts normal dietary advice, and quotes the Royal College of Psychiatrists of London as saying that 'for women, more than 14 alcoholic units, or two bottles of champagne a week, can contribute to death from liver disease, cancer of the gullet and pancreas, and a 47 per cent increased likelihood of a fatal fall'.

2 A.L. Stewart and R.H. Brook (1983) 'Effects of being overweight', *American Journal of Public Health* 73, 2: 171–7.

3 R.W. Jeffery, A.R. Folsom, R.V. Luepker, D.R. Jacobs, R.F. Gillum, H.L. Taylor, and H. Blackburn (1984) 'Prevalence of overweight and weight loss behavior in a metropolitan adult population: the Minnesota heart survey experience', *American Journal of Public Health* 74, 4: 349–52.

4 *Medical and Health Care Books and Serials in Print: An Index to Literature in the Health Sciences*, vol. 1 (1986) New York: Bowker.

5 *British Rate and Data* 1966, 1976, 1986.

6 *Which Way to Slim* (1978) London: Consumers' Association.

7 Cited by E.S. Parham, V.L. Frigo, and A.H. Perkins (1982) 'Weight control as portrayed in popular magazines', *Journal of Nutrition Education* 14, 4: 153–6.

8 K.K. Grunewald (1985) 'Weight control in young college women: who are the dieters? *Research* 85, 11: 1445–50.

9 E.S. Parham, S.L. King, M.L. Bedell, and S. Martersteck (1986) 'Weight control content of women's magazines: bias and accuracy', *International Journal of Obesity* 10: 19–27.

Dr Parham and her colleagues analysed the content of sixty-seven articles on weight control from thirty-seven popular magazines available on news-stands in Illinois in 1982. These magazines included top-selling magazines, diet and exercise magazines, women's magazines, and 'teen' magazines. Most of the articles depicted achieving normal weight as relatively hard and slow, but likely. Only 11 per cent of the articles were judged as generally pessimistic.

10 S. Schachter (1982) 'Recidivism and self-cure of smoking and obesity', *American Psychologist* 37, 4: 436–44.

11 Jeffery *et al.* (1984) op. cit.

12 A. Eyton (1987) 'Self-help lay groups', *Body Weight Control: The Physiology, Treatment and Prevention of Obesity*, London: Churchill Livingstone, p. 140.

13 Eyton (1987) op. cit., p. 145.

14 F.R. Volkmar, A.J. Stunkard, J. Woolston, and R.A. Bailey (1981) 'High attrition rates in commercial weight reduction programs', *Archives of Internal Medicine*, 141: 426–8.

15 S. Levy, J.P. Pearce, N. Dembecki, and A. Cripps (1986) 'Self-help group behavioural treatment for obesity: an evaluation of weight control workshops', *Medical Journal of Australia* 145: 436–8.

16 M. Ashwell and J.S. Garrow (1978) 'A survey of three slimming and weight control organisations in the U.K.', *Nutrition* 29: 347–56.

17 D. Craddock (1973) *Obesity and its Management*, Edinburgh and London: Churchill Livingstone.

18 G. Bennett (1987) 'Behaviour therapy in the treatment of obesity', in R.A. Boakes, M.J. Burton, and D.A. Popplewell (eds) *Eating Habits: Food, Physiology and Learned Behaviour*, Chichester and New York: John Wiley, p. 50.

19 G.K. Simpson, V.E. Abernethy, and J.F. Munro (1987) 'Treatment with drugs' in A.E. Bender and L.J. Brookes (eds) *Body Weight Control: The Physiology, Clinical Treatment and Prevention of Obesity*, Edinburgh and London: Churchill Livingstone, pp. 117–26.

20 Simpson *et al.* (1987) op. cit.

21 R.B. Stuart, C. Mitchell, and J. Jensen (1981) 'Therapeutic options in the management of obesity', in C. Prokop and L. Bradley (eds) *Medical Psychology: Contributions to Behavioural Medicine*, New York: Academic Press.

22 People who do wish to find themselves a therapist to help with a psychological problem should bear in mind the following points. With regard to hypnotists: in Britain, anyone can set themselves up as a hypnotherapist or therapist without any qualifications or training. People who advertise themselves in newspapers are usually lay therapists who may have trained with private organizations. However, there is no such profession as 'hypnotherapist' and no qualification in 'hypnotherapy' recognized by the Health Service or academic institutions. Hypnosis may be carried out by people such as medical doctors, dentists or psychologists who are trained in the technique in addition to their own profession. There are two relevant professional societies: The British Society of Experimental and Clinical Hypnosis (Hon. Secretary Michael Heap, Psychology Department, Middlewood Hospital, Sheffield S6 1TP); and the British Society of Medical and

Dental Hypnosis (P.O. Box 6, Ashtead, Surrey KT21 2HJ).
With regard to psychologists: from mid-1989 the British Psychological Society will have a Register of Chartered Psychologists containing the names of properly trained psychologists, who will be entitled to use the abbreviation 'C. Psychol.' after their name. The register is non-statutory, which means that psychologists do not have to register by law, but that the public can be sure that those people who are registered are fully qualified in their own field of psychology and in accordance with their code of conduct should not lay claim to skills they do not have. After August 1989 there should be a copy of the register available in local libraries.

The address of the British Psychological Society is: St. Andrew's House, 48 Princess Road East, Leicester LE1 7DR.

23 As the emphasis of this book is on psychological rather than nutritional aspects of dieting, it is not intended to attempt to make detailed recommendations about foods that should be used or avoided. There is a plethora of books detailing the nutritional requirements of reducing diets. The chief problem, however, facing the would-be dieter is to know how to recognize the sound as opposed to the ridiculous, often misleading, advice. Readers seeking further information might wish to look at one of the following references: P. Nicholas and J. Dwyer (1986) 'Diets for weight reduction: nutritional considerations', in *Handbook of Eating Disorders: Physiology, Psychology and Treatment of Obesity, Anorexia and Bulimia* K.D. Brownell and J.P. Foreyt (eds) New York: Basic Books, pp. 122–44.
British Dietetic Association (1985) *The Great British Diet*, London: Century Publishing.
With regard to the very low-calorie diets now available in drink form from several companies, specialists in both the United States and Britain have seriously questioned the sense and the safety of their use without close medical supervision and in any but the most severely overweight people. For an authoritative report and critique on very low-calorie diets see: Department of Health and Social Security Report on Health and Social Subjects number 31, 'The Use of Very Low Calorie Diets in Obesity', London: Her Majesty's Stationery Office.

24 Consumers' Association (1978) op. cit., p. 39.

25 Consumers' Association (1978) op. cit.

26 A. Grimsmo, G. Helgesen, and C. Borchgrevink (1981) 'Short-term and long-term effects of lay groups on weight reduction', *British Medical Journal* 283: 1093–5.

27 M. Ashwell and J.S. Garrow (1978) op. cit.

2 WHY DIET?

1 J.S. Garrow (1981) *Treat Obesity Seriously: A Clinical Manual*, Edinburgh and London: Churchill Livingstone, p. 18.
2 W.P.T. James (1987) 'Being overweight: a working definition', in A.E. Bender and L.J. Brookes (eds) *Body Weight Control: The Physiology, Clinical Treatment and Prevention of Obesity*, Edinburgh, London, Melbourne, and New York: Churchill Livingstone, pp. 90–106.

> In India the average weight of the adult male approximates to the lowest of the weights considered appropriate for optimal health in Britain. Yet one could argue that in India a man who is potentially subject to periodic famines might live longer by virtue of having a greater body weight and body fat mass than a male living in the United Kingdom. Furthermore, it has been suggested that obese adults who become obese in developing countries, e.g. Southern Africa, may have fewer complications associated with obesity for dietary or other, e.g. genetic, reasons. (p. 90)

3 Obesity is not the same as overweight. It is possible to weigh more than average for other reasons than having a high proportion of fat in the body, for example, some athletes weigh more because they carry more muscle than other people.

> G.A. Bray (1986) 'Effects of obesity on health and happiness', in K.D. Brownell and J.P. Foreyt (eds) *Handbook of Eating Disorders: Physiology, Psychology and Treatment of Obesity, Anorexia and Bulimia*, New York: Basic Books, pp. 3–44.

4 Metropolitan Life Insurance Company, New York (1960) 'Mortality among overweight men and women', *Statistical Bulletin* 4, pt 1.

> G.A. Bray (1979) 'Obesity in America' in *Proceedings of the 2nd Fogarty International Centre Conference on Obesity No. 79*, Washington DC: US Department of Health Education and Welfare.

The Metropolitan Life Insurance Company published its figures on weights and heights for a wide range of people. They derived the table from weights associated with the lowest mortality rates among the people insured with them. One criticism of such figures has been that people who choose to insure their lives are not representative of the population as a whole. Another criticism has been that the weights were divided for the sake of convenience into three frame sizes – 'small', 'medium', and 'large'; these figures can often be seen reproduced in the popular slimming press. In fact there is no justification for dividing the weights arbitrarily in this way and the 1979 revision has no separate categorization of individuals into frame size.

5 James (1987) op. cit., p. 90.
6 Bray (1986) op. cit., p. 4.
7 J.S. Garrow (1979) 'Weight penalties, *British Medical Journal* 2: 1171–2.

8 'Obesity: a report of the Royal College of Physicians' (1983) *Journal of the Royal College of Physicians of London* 17, 1: 21.
9 Bray (1986) op. cit., p. 29.
10 B.T. Burton, W.R. Foster, J. Hirsch, and T.B. Van Itallie (1985) 'Health implications of obesity: an NIH consensus development conference', *International Journal of Obesity* 9: 155–69.
11 Burton *et al.* (1985) op. cit., p. 158.
12 Bray (1986) op. cit., pp. 16–17.
13 James (1987) op. cit., p. 99.
14 One study of a health care programme in California reported that thin male and female current cigarette smokers were at increased risk of mortality compared with average weight smokers. Thinness itself was not associated with increased mortality in ex-smokers or in people who had never smoked.
   S. Sidney, G. Friedman, and A.B. Siegelaub (1987) 'Thinness and mortality', *American Journal of Public Health* 77, pt 3: 317–22.
15 E.A. Lew and E.A. Garfinkel (1979) 'Variations in mortality by weight among 750,000 men and women', *Journal of Chronic Diseases* 32: 563–76.
   American Cancer Society Study, cited by Bray (1986) op. cit.
16 Body Mass Index (BMI) is weight (in kilograms) divided by height (in metres) squared, i.e. 75/(1.64 x 1.64).
17 'Obesity: a report of the Royal College of Physicians' (1983) *Journal of the Royal College of Physicians of London* 17, 1: 20.
18 Bray (1986) op. cit., p. 17.
19 S. Gilbert (1986) *Pathology of Eating: Psychology and Treatment*, Routledge & Kegan Paul, pp. 6–7.
20 S.A. Richardson, A.H. Hastorf, N. Goodman, and S.M. Dornbusch (1961) 'Cultural uniformity in reaction to physical disabilities', *American Sociological Review* 90: 44–51.
21 J.R. Staffieri (1967) 'A study of social stereotype of body image in children', *Journal of Personality and Social Psychology* 7: 101–4.
22 S.C. Wooley (1987) 'Psychological and social aspects of obesity', in A.E. Bender and L.J. Brookes (eds) *Body Weight Control*, Edinburgh, London, Melbourne, and New York: Churchill Livingstone, pp. 81–9.
23 G.L. Maddox (1968) 'Overweight as social deviance and disability', *Journal of Health and Social Behavior* 9: 287–98.
24 H. Canning and J. Mayer (1966) 'Obesity: its possible effect on college acceptance', *New England Journal of Medicine* 275, 1172–4.
25 A group of health care students in an American college was shown pictures of male and female 'clients' of different weights but with the same history attached to the pictures. The students had to say what they thought was most likely to happen to the imaginary 'clients' and choose from a range of service delivery options for them. When given identical information, the students had more positive attitudes towards a 'client' who was shown as normal weight than to one shown as obese. When shown as obese, the 'client' was more likely

to be recommended for a dependent role – counselling or a sheltered
workshop – and less likely to be funded for college training.

    S.P. Kaplan (1984) 'Rehabilitation counseling students' perceptions
of obese male and female clients', *Rehabilitation Counseling Bulletin*
27: pt 3: 172–81.

26 D.M. Garner, P.E. Garfinkel, and M.P. Olmstead (1983) 'An
overview of sociocultural factors in the development of anorexia
nervosa', in P.L. Darby, P.E. Garfinkel, D.M. Garner, and D.V.
Coscina (eds) *Anorexia Nervosa: Recent Developments in Research*,
New York: Alan R. Liss, pp. 65–82.

27 D.M. Garner and P.E. Garfinkel (1980) 'Socio-cultural factors in the
development of anorexia nervosa', *Psychological Medicine* 19, pt 4:
647–56.

28 L. Kurman, 'An analysis of messages concerning food, eating
behaviours, and ideal body-image on prime-time American network
television', *Dissertation Abstract*, cited by Garner *et al.* (1983) op.
cit.

29 All the examples in the book are true, but I have modified situations
and given the characters fictitious names to protect their privacy.

30 *Which Way to Slim* (1978) London: Consumers' Association.

31 J.C. Seidell, K.C. Bakx, P. Deurenberg, J. Burema, J.G.A.J.
Hautvast, and F.J.A. Huygen (1986) 'The relation between
overweight and subjective health according to age, social class,
slimming behavior and smoking habits in Dutch adults', *American
Journal of Public Health* 76, 12: 1410–15.

3 CAUSES OF OBESITY

1 M. Stock and N. Rothwell (1982) *Obesity and Leanness: Basic
Aspects*, London: John Libbey, p. 79.

2 'Obesity: a report of the Royal College of Physicians' (1983) *Journal
of the Royal College of Physicians of London* 17, 1: 25.

3 T.B. Van Itallie and C.E. Woteki (1987) 'Who gets fat?' in A.E.
Bender and L.J. Brookes (eds) *Body Weight Control*, Edinburgh,
London, Melbourne, and New York: Churchill Livingstone, pp. 50–1.

4 S.M. Garn, S.M. Bailey, M.A. Solomon, and P.J. Hopkins (1981)
'Effect of remaining family members on fatness prediction', *American
Journal of Clinical Nutrition*, 34: 148–53.

5 S.M. Garn (1986) 'Family-line and socioeconomic factors in fatness
and obesity', *Nutrition Reviews* 44, 12: 381–6.

6 E. Mason (1970) 'Obesity in pet dogs', *Veterinary Research* 86:
612–16.

7 L. Sjostrom (1980) 'Fat cells and body weight', in A. Stunkard (ed.)
Obesity, Eastbourne and Philadelphia: W.B. Saunders, p. 93.

8 Stock and Rothwell (1982) op. cit., p. 11; see also J.S. Garrow
(1981) *Treat Obesity Seriously: A Clinical Manual*, Edinburgh:
Churchill Livingstone, for detailed explanations of the physiology of
obesity and of energy balance.

9 'Obesity: a report of the Royal College of Physicians' (1983) *Journal of the Royal College of Physicians of London* 17, 1: 37.

10 K. Brownell and A.J. Stunkard (1980) 'Physical activity in the development and control of obesity', in A.J. Stunkard (ed.) *Obesity*, Eastbourne and Philadelphia: W.B. Saunders, p. 301.

11 J.S. Garrow (1981) *Treat Obesity Seriously: A Clinical Manual*, Edinburgh: Churchill Livingstone, p. 155.

12 L.E. Braitman, E.V. Adlin, and J.L. Stanton, jun. (1985) 'Obesity and caloric intake: the national health and nutrition examination survey of 1971–1975 (HANES I)', *Journal of Chronic Diseases* 18, 9: 727–32.

13 L. Spitzer and J. Rodin (1981) 'Human eating behavior: a critical review of studies in normal weight and overweight individuals', *Appetite: Journal for Intake Research* 2, 293–329.

14 A.J. Stunkard and A. Mazer (1978) 'Smorgasbord and obesity', *Psychosomatic Medicine* 40, 2: 173–5.

15 W.M. Beneke and C.H. Davis (1985) 'Relationship of hunger, use of a shopping list and obesity to food purchases', *International Journal of Obesity* 9: 391–9.

16 H. Bruch (1974) *Eating Disorders: Anorexia, Obesity and the Person Within*, London and Boston, Mass: Routledge & Kegan Paul.

4 WHAT IS HUNGER? OR 'WHY CAN'T I JUST STOP EATING WHEN I WANT TO?'

1 S. Orbach (1978) *Fat is a Feminist Issue: The Anti-Diet Guide to Permanent Weight Loss*, New York and London: Paddington Press.

2 S. Hashim and T.B. Van Itallie (1965) 'Studies in normal and obese subjects with a monitored food dispensing device', *Annals of the New York Academy of Science* 131, Art. 1: 654–61.

3 S.C. Wooley (1972) 'Physiologic versus cognitive factors in short term food regulation in the obese and nonobese', *Psychosomatic Medicine* 34, 1: 62–8.

4 For a detailed account of this work, see B.J. Rolls, E.T. Rolls, and E.A. Rowe (1982) 'The influence of variety on human food selection and intake', in L.M. Barker (ed.) *The Psychobiology of Human Food Selection*, Westport, Conn: Avi Publishing, pp. 101–22.

5 For a fascinating and highly detailed historical and social survey of food and cuisine, see S. Mennell (1985) *All Manners of Food: Eating and Taste in England and France from the Middle Ages to the Present*, Oxford and New York: Blackwell.

6 Mennell (1985) op. cit., p. 31.

7 J. Hankin, D. Reed, D. Labarthe, M. Nichaman, and R. Stallones (1970) 'Dietary and disease patterns among Micronesians', *American Journal of Clinical Nutrition* 23: 346–57.

8 L.L. Birch, S.I. Zimmerman, and H. Hind (1980) 'The influence of social-affective context on the formation of children's food preferences', *Child Development* 51, pt 3: 856–61.

9 L.L. Birch, D.W. Marlin, and J. Rotter (1984) 'Eating as the "means" activity in a contingency: effects on young children's food preference', *Child Development* 55, pt 2: 431–9.
10 G.K. Beauchamp and M. Moran (1982) 'Dietary experience and sweet taste preference in human infants', *Appetite: Journal for Intake Research* 3, pt 2: 139–52.
11 J.E. Blundell and A.J. Hill (1985) 'Analysis of hunger: interrelationships with palatability, nutrient composition and eating', in J. Hirsch and T.B. Van Itallie (eds) *Recent Advances in Obesity Research: IV*, London and Paris: John Libbey, pp. 118–29.
12 A. Drenowski and M.R.C. Greenwood (1983) 'Cream and sugar: human preferences for high-fat foods', *Physiology and Behavior* 30: 629–33.
13 S. Schachter (1968) 'Obesity and eating', *Science* 161: 751–6.
14 For a summary of research in this area, see C.P. Herman and J. Polivy (1980) 'Restrained eating', in A.J. Stunkard (ed.) *Obesity*, Eastbourne and Philadelphia: W.B. Saunders, pp. 208–25.

5 SUCCESSFUL SLIMMING

1 N. Allon (1975) 'Fat is a dirty word: fat as a sociological and social problem', in A.N. Howard (ed.) *Recent Advances in Obesity Research: 1*, London: Newman Publishing, pp. 244–7.
  Natalie Allon spent four years observing and taking part in a slimming organization in New York. In her experience the slimmers were socialized into perceiving 'fat' as a dirty word and overweight as 'sinful deviation'.
2 G. Cannon and H. Einzig (1983) *Dieting Makes You Fat*, London: Century Publishing, pp. 194–7.
3 E.A. Baanders-van Halewijn, Y.W. Choy, J. Van Uitert, and F. de Waard (1984) 'The Cordon Study of weight reduction based on behaviour modification', *International Journal of Obesity* 8, pt 2: 161–70.
4 See 'The slob's diet', *Slimming* magazine, January/February 1987, p. 43.
5 J.G. Douglas, M.J. Ford, and J.F. Munro (1981) 'Patient motivation and predicting outcome in a hospital obesity clinic', *International Journal of Obesity* 5: 33–8.
6 For a more detailed discussion see S. Gilbert (1986) *Pathology of Eating: Psychology and Treatment*, London and Boston, Mass: Routledge & Kegan Paul, pp. 174–5.
7 See for example, K.D. Brownell, C.L. Heckerman, R.J. Westlake, S.C. Hayes, and P.M. Monti (1978) 'The effect of couples training and partner co-operativeness in the behavioural treatment of obesity', *Behaviour Research and Therapy* 16: 323–33.
8 A.Z. Belko, M. Van Loan, T.F. Barbieri, and P. Mayclin (1986) 'Diet, exercise, weight loss, and energy expenditure in moderately overweight women', *International Journal of Obesity* 11: 93–104.

9 J.S. Stern (1984) 'Is obesity a disease of inactivity?', *Research Publication of the Association of Research into Nervous and Mental Diseases* 62, 131-9.
10 J.S. Garrow (1987) 'Effect of exercise on obesity', *Acta Medica Scandinavica Supplement* 711: 67-73.
11 Garrow (1987) op. cit., p. 71.
12 R.E. Frisch, G. Wyshak, N.L. Albright *et al.* (1985) 'Lower prevalence of breast cancer and cancers of the reproductive system among former college athletes compared to non-athletes', *British Journal of Cancer* 52: 885-91.
13 Cannon and Einzig (1983) op. cit., pp. 216-17.

6 THE DARK SIDE OF DIETING

1 See C. Cummings, J.R. Gordon, and G.A. Marlatt (1980) 'Relapse: prevention and prediction', in W.R. Miller (ed.) *The Addictive Behaviors: Treatment of Alcoholism, Drug Abuse and Obesity*, Oxford: Pergamon, pp. 291-322.
2 J.S. Garrow (1981) *Treat Obesity Seriously: A Clinical Manual*, Edinburgh and London: Churchill Livingstone, p. 22.
3 C.W. Calloway and C. Pemberton (1983) 'Relationship of basal metabolic rates to meal eating patterns', Poster presentation at International Congress of Obesity in New York.
4 A. Keys, J. Brozek, A. Henschel, O. Mickelson, and H.L. Taylor (1950) *The Biology of Human Starvation*, Minneapolis: University of Minnesota Press.
5 D.M. Zuckerman, A. Colby, N.C. Ware, and J.S. Lagerson (1986) 'The prevalence of bulimia among college students', *American Journal of Public Health* 76, pt 9: 1135-7.
6 P.J. Cooper, G. Waterman, and C.G. Fairburn (1984) 'Women with eating problems: a community survey', *British Journal of Clinical Psychology* 23: 45-52.
7 Some people become emaciated initially not through excessive dieting but simply through inability to eat, perhaps as a result of a long period of great unhappiness or through a fear of possible nausea or discomfort when they do eat. It can be very difficult to make the distinction between people with true anorexia nervosa, who often deny their wish to be slim and do not admit to hunger, and these people.
8 H. Bruch (1974) *Eating Disorders: Anorexia, Obesity and the Person Within*, London and Boston, Mass: Routledge & Kegan Paul.
9 The criteria for diagnosing anorexia nervosa as a psychiatric disorder vary between medical authorities. Generally the criterion of at least 25 per cent of matched population mean weight (the average weight for height of a person of the same height and sex) is required; but weight loss can vary between individuals and many anorexics weigh as little as 65 per cent of MPMW or less.

  See also American Psychiatric Association (1987) *Diagnostic and Statistical Manual of Mental Disorders* (revised), 4th edn, Washington DC.

10 A.H. Crisp, L.K.G. Hsu, B. Harding, and J. Hartshorn (1980) 'Clinical features of anorexia nervosa: a study of a consecutive series of 102 female patients', *Journal of Psychosomatic Research* 24: 179-91.
11 G.M. Rodin, D. Daneman, L.E. Johnson, A. Kenshole, and P. Garfinkel (1985) 'Anorexia nervosa and bulimia in female adolescents with insulin dependent diabetes mellitus: a systematic study', *Journal of Psychiatric Research* 19, pts 2 and 3: 381-4.
12 D.M. Garner and P.E. Garfinkel (1980) 'Sociocultural factors in the development of anorexia nervosa', *Psychological Medicine* 19, pt 4: 647-56.
13 E.J. Button and A. Whitehouse (1981) 'Subclinical anorexia nervosa', *Psychological Medicine* 11, pt 3: 509-16.
14 G.I. Szmukler, I. Eisler, C. Gillies, and M.E. Hayward (1985) 'The implications of anorexia nervosa in a ballet school', *Journal of Psychiatric Research* 19, pts 2 and 3: 177-81.
15 A. Fursland (1987) 'Eve was framed: food and sex and women's shame' in M. Lawrence (ed.) *Fed Up and Hungry: Women, Oppression, and Food*, London: Women's Press, p. 16.

7 EATING TO LIVE

1 A Discussion Paper on Proposals for Nutritional Guidelines for Health Education in Britain, prepared for the National Advisory Committee on Nutrition Education (NACNE) by an *ad hoc* working party under the chairmanship of Professor W.P.T. James (1983) London: Health Education Council. NACNE was set up initially to summarize all the available information on eating and health and produce a report which could set out guidelines for the health professionals and organizations with the aim of improving the nation's eating habits. The report was based on the conclusions of eight reports of expert committees including the DHSS and the Royal College of Physicians set up previously by the government. In fact when it came to publication there was a great deal of controversy, with some of the members of NACNE declining to indicate their agreement with the report and its recommendations. There were suggestions made that the report was in conflict with the interests of the food industry, represented on the committee.

An interesting summary of the story of the report is given in C. Walker and G. Cannon (1985) *The Food Scandal*, London: Century Publishing. This book describes the main recommendations of the report and also gives some explanations for the reasoning behind it. In addition it gives useful advice about how to put the recommendations into practice and avoid falling into the trap of eating food which is poor in nutritional value by explaining how foods are processed and the meanings of labels in food packaging.
2 See Dr Juliet Gray (1986) *Food Intolerance: Fact and Fiction*, London: Grafton Books. Subtitled 'A practical guide to allergy and

other food reactions', this book aims to clear up misunderstandings about the subject of food allergy and offer advice to sufferers. It is based on a report of the Royal College of Physicians with the British Nutrition Foundation, entitled 'Food intolerance and food aversion' and published in April 1984, *Journal of the Royal College of Physicians of London* 18, 2.

3 The McGovern Report (1977) *Dietary Goals for the United States*, a report of a United States Senate Committee.

4 About half the fats we eat are saturated fats. These are mainly solid in form and come mainly from animals but also from coconut oil and palm oil. Polyunsaturated fats are mostly liquid in their natural form and are of vegetable origin (e.g. olive oil, sunflower oil) and fish origin.

5 Processed foods include frozen and tinned foods, and not all are bad. See: *Guide to Healthy Eating*, free from the Health Education Authority.

6 J.W. Anderson (1986) 'Fiber and health: an overview', *American Journal of Gastroenterology* 81, 10: 892-7.

7 British Dietetic Association (1985) *The Great British Diet*, London: Century Publishing.

8 L. Birch (1987) 'The acquisition of food acceptance patterns in children', in R.A. Boakes, M.J. Burton, and D.A. Popplewell (eds) *Eating Habits: Food, Physiology and Learned Behaviour*, Chichester and New York: John Wiley, pp. 107-30.

9 J. Dunn (1980) 'Feeding and sleeping', in M. Rutter (ed.) *Scientific Foundations of Developmental Psychiatry*, London: Heinemann, pp. 119-28.

10 US Government report cited by Birch (1987) op. cit., p. 126.

11 Birch (1987) op. cit., pp. 123-4. Ms Birch cites research that suggests that children are more likely to taste a food they have not had before if they see an adult eating it than if the adult simply offers it to them.

8 COPING WITH A DIET 1: DEFINING THE PROBLEM

1 S. Orbach (1978) *Fat is a Feminist Issue*, New York and London: Paddington Press, pp. 139-40.

2 There are several questionnaires in existence, some of them asking questions along similar lines. In order for a questionnaire to be regarded as a reliable measure of a particular set of feelings or behaviours, it has to undergo rigorous research, whereby it is administered to as many as a hundred or more people and the answers are examined together with other information about those people. I have compiled this questionnaire in an attempt to reflect current explanations of eating and overeating and as a stimulus to thinking about individual eating styles. In common with most questionnaires published in books and magazines, it has no status as a measuring instrument and you should not assume that it is necessarily

a valid or reliable measure of the extent of an eating problem or that it can be used to compare one person with another.

9 COPING WITH A DIET 2: PLANNING FOR CHANGE

1 R.B. Stuart and B. Davis (1972) *Slim Chance in a Fat World: Behavioral Control of Obesity*, Champaign, Ill: Research Press.
2 L.H. Epstein, R.R. Wing, R. Koeske, and A. Valoski (1987) 'Long-term effects of family based treatment of childhood obesity', *Journal of Consulting and Clinical Psychology* 55, 1: 91–5.
3 See also L.H. Epstein and M.S. Squires (1988) *The Stop-Light Diet for Children: An Eight-Week Program for Parents and Children*, Boston: Little, Brown, and Company.
4 It may help you to read some more about how to be assertive. See A. Dickson (1982) *A Woman in Your Own Right*, London: Quartet Books; M.J. Smith (1975) *When I Say No, I Feel Guilty*, New York, London and Toronto: Bantam.
5 For further information about coping with stress and learning how to relax see K. Hambly (1983) *Overcoming Tension*, London: Sheldon Press; D. Meichenbaum (1983) *Coping with Stress*, London: Century Publishing.

10 ALTERNATIVES TO WILL-POWER

1 A.T. Beck, A.J. Rush, B.F. Shaw, and G. Emery (1976) *Cognitive Therapy of Depression*, New York: John Wiley.
  For an excellent self-help approach to depression, see D. Burns (1981) *Feeling Good: The New Mood Therapy*, New York: Signet.
  For a guide to getting help for psychological problems (in Britain) see: H. Edwards, (1987) *Psychological Problems: Who Can Help?*, British Psychological Society and Methuen.

INDEX

For Product Safety Concerns and Information please contact our EU representative GPSR@taylorandfrancis.com Taylor & Francis Verlag GmbH, Kaufingerstraße 24, 80331 München, Germany

Printed and bound by CPI Group (UK) Ltd, Croydon, CR0 4YY
01/05/2025
01858546-0001